The EVERYTHING® Diabetes Book

Dear Reader:

I married into diabetes, so to speak. My father-in-law has had type 2 for several decades, controlled first by oral medications and now by insulin. But my first brush with the disease occurred when I was about twelve and saw a younger relative of mine, a "juvenile diabetic" as I was quietly told at the time, deftly administer an insulin injection. I remember both marveling at his bravery and being a little afraid that I'd catch whatever it was he had. Silence does a lot to fuel the imagination.

Today we talk about diabetes more openly, but much misinformation and mystery still surrounds type 1, type 2, and gestational diabetes. I receive dozens of e-mails each week from patients and family thrown into the bewildering world of diabetes—some with just a prescription and a handshake—looking for a way to get their heads and hearts around this life-altering disease. For that reason, I wrote *The Everything® Diabetes Book* as both a user-friendly road map to the basics of diabetes and its treatment and as a guide to integrating control into your daily routine—to live life with diabetes, and not for it.

Paula Ford-Martin

The EVERYTHING® Series

Editorial

Publishing Director	Gary M. Krebs
Managing Editor	Kate McBride
Copy Chief	Laura MacLaughlin
Acquisitions Editor	Eric M. Hall
Development Editor	Julie Gutin
Production Editor	Khrysti Nazzaro

Production

Production Director	Susan Beale
Production Manager	Michelle Roy Kelly
Series Designers	Daria Perreault Colleen Cunningham
Cover Design	Paul Beatrice Frank Rivera
Layout and Graphics	Colleen Cunningham Rachael Eiben Michelle Roy Kelly Daria Perreault Erin Ring
Series Cover Artist	Barry Littmann
Interior Illustrator	Eric Andrews

THE EVERYTHING® DIABETES BOOK

From diagnosis and diet to insulin and exercise, all you need to live a healthy, active life

Paula Ford-Martin with Ian Blumer, M.D.

Adams Media
Avon, Massachusetts

For Bob—Superdad, politico, and all around great guy.

An Everything® Series Book.

Published by Adams Media, an F+W Publications Company
57 Littlefield Street, Avon, MA 02322 U.S.A
www.adamsmedia.com

ISBN: 1-58062-981-4
Printed in the United States of America.

J I H G F E D C

Library of Congress Cataloging-in-Publication Data
Ford-Martin, Paula.
The everything diabetes book / Paula Ford-Martin, with Ian Blumer.
p. cm.
(An everything series book)
ISBN 1-58062-981-4
1. Diabetes–Popular works. I. Blumer, Ian. II. Title.
III. Series: Everything series.
RC660.4.F67 2003
616.4'62–dc21 2003014700

The Everything® Diabetes Book is intended as a reference volume only, not as a medical manual. In light of the complex, individual, and specific nature of health problems, this book is not intended to replace professional medical advice. The ideas, procedures, and suggestions in this book are intended to supplement, not replace, the advice of a trained medical professional. Consult your physician before adopting the suggestions in this book, as well as about any condition that may require diagnosis or medical attention. The authors and publisher disclaim any liability arising directly or indirectly from the use of this book.

This book is available at quantity discounts for bulk purchases.
For information, call 1-800-872-5627.

Contents

Acknowledgments

My heartfelt thanks to Ian Blumer, M.D., whose knowledge, experience, and terrific sense of humor made writing this book a pleasure. And to those who made writing it a privilege—thanks to Marcie, Andrea, Harvie, Sandi, Char, Bev, and all the other "regulars" at the About Diabetes forum. Your courage, compassion, and insight have helped so many—including me. Finally, thanks to Barb Doyen and Eric Hall, encouragement and patience personified.

Top Ten Things You Should Know
About Diabetes

1. Eating sugar does not cause diabetes. And contrary to popular belief, people with diabetes can eat sugar in moderation, as long as it's figured in to their overall meal plans.
2. The terms "insulin-dependent" (type 1) and "non-insulin-dependent" (type 2) diabetes are obsolete. People with type 2 diabetes do require insulin sometimes.
3. Adults can develop "juvenile" (type 1) diabetes and kids can develop "adult-onset" (type 2) diabetes.
4. Having "a touch" of diabetes is like being "a touch" pregnant. There is no such thing as borderline diabetes.
5. There is no "diabetic diet," only a new, healthier way of eating.
6. Attending a diabetes education class and meeting with a registered dietitian are two of the most important ways you can start controlling your diabetes.
7. People with diabetes can work out and play sports. Exercise lowers blood glucose levels and is an important component of good diabetes management.
8. Diabetes is not a death sentence, but it can lead to serious, life-altering and life-threatening complications if ignored.
9. Checking yourself frequently with a home blood glucose monitor can help prevent blood sugar emergencies and is an invaluable tool for learning how food and medication affect your disease.
10. People with diabetes—both adults and children—are protected against discrimination in the workplace and at school by a number of federal laws.

Introduction

▶IF YOU'VE PICKED UP THIS BOOK, chances are that diabetes has touched your life or the life of someone close to you. Whatever the manifestation—type 1, type 2, or gestational—diabetes can be a frightening and personally devastating diagnosis. Fortunately, patient knowledge and action are probably the two most important components to staying on top of this disease.

A key phrase in the lexicon of diabetes care is *good control.* For those new to the topic, good control means keeping your blood glucose, or blood sugar, in a range at or close to normal through diet, exercise, and/or medication. Control is the key to managing diabetes mentally as well as physically. The power is in your hands to make a difference in how diabetes affects your life.

Many people feel out of control of their diabetes. Some ignore it completely in a fog of denial. Others follow medical instructions to the letter yet never ask questions of their doctor or provide any feedback. The latter may get a handle on their blood glucose levels, but are so miserable it hardly matters.

Managing diabetes requires education, dedication, and a certain doggedness of character. Most important, it requires a commitment to being a leader, not a follower, in your own health care. Surrounding yourself with good people—endocrinologists, internists, certified diabetes educators, registered dietitians, and more—is an excellent start. But it takes more than a crack medical team to control diabetes. Even the best team will falter without a coach, and that leader is you. Playing an active role in your own health care is essential to staying both healthy and happy.

Uncontrolled blood glucose levels wreck havoc on the body, short-circuiting just about every system over time if not managed properly. Heart disease, stroke, high blood pressure, retinopathy, kidney disease, and nerve damage are just a few of the complications that diabetes leaves in its wake. This is why educating yourself about the intricacies of glucose control—through diet, exercise, medication, lifestyle, and more—is so very essential.

Medical breakthroughs like islet cell transplantation, advances in glucose monitoring technologies and new oral medications and insulin formulations have drastically improved the quality of life for all people with diabetes, but there is still no cure for the disease. Until there is, staying current on developments in diabetes management, communicating with your health care team, and staying on top of self-care through positive lifestyle choices are absolutely essential to wellness. *The Everything® Diabetes Book* was designed to be your reference partner in staying healthy with diabetes.

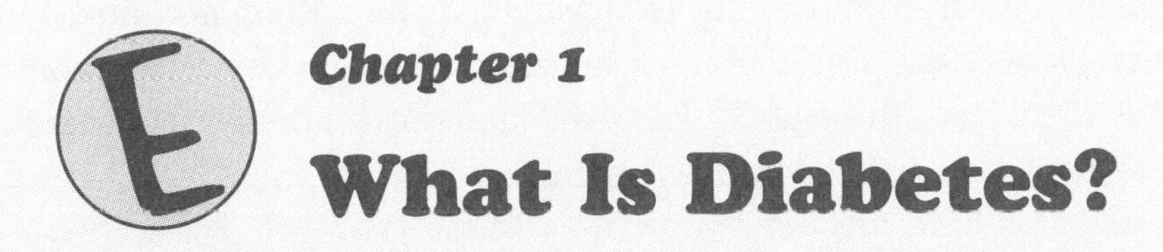

Chapter 1

What Is Diabetes?

Diabetes mellitus comes in many flavors—type 1, type 2, gestational, and variations such as maturity-onset diabetes in the young (MODY) and latent autoimmune diabetes of adulthood (LADA). What all of these disorders have in common is an inherent inability to self-regulate the levels of blood glucose—or cellular fuel—in the body.

A Growing Problem

The U.S. Centers for Disease Control has called diabetes "an emerging epidemic." The statistics say it all. In 2002, the National Institutes of Health and the CDC put the number of U.S. residents diagnosed with diabetes at a staggering 17 million. That's about 10 percent of the estimated 170 million people suffering from diabetes worldwide. Another 16 million people in the United States have prediabetes, or impaired glucose tolerance, a condition that is a precursor to type 2 diabetes. Many remain dangerously unaware of the condition and the consequences.

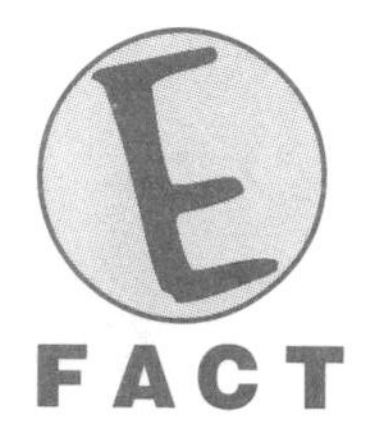

FACT

Type 2 diabetes accounts for 90 to 95 percent of the total diabetes population in the United States and is the sixth leading cause of death in America. But moderate levels of regular physical activity and a healthy diet can cut a person's chance of developing type 2 by up to 60 percent.

In addition to the physical and emotional toll it exacts, diabetes also comes with an enormous price tag. According to the American Diabetes Association (ADA), the disease costs Americans $132 billion annually in medical expenses and lost productivity. And it isn't just diabetes that's running up the tab. Over $24 billion of those annual costs are for expenses related to chronic diabetic complications.

The Endocrine System

Diabetes mellitus is classified as a disease of the endocrine system. The endocrine system is composed of glands that secrete the hormones that travel through the circulatory system to regulate metabolism, growth, sexual development, and reproduction. When one of these pivotal glands—the adrenals, the thyroid and parathyroid, the thymus, the pituitary, testes, ovaries, and the pancreas—secretes either too little or too much of a hormone, the entire body can be thrown off balance.

The Pancreas and Liver

One of the endocrine glands, the pancreas, actually pulls double duty as a digestive organ. Sitting behind the stomach, the spongy pancreas secretes both digestive enzymes and endocrine hormones. It is long and tapered with a thicker bottom end (or head), which is cradled in the downward curve of the duodenum–a part of the small intestine or bowel. The long end (or tail) of the pancreas extends up behind the stomach toward the spleen (see figure on page 5). A main duct, or channel, connects the pancreas to the duodenum.

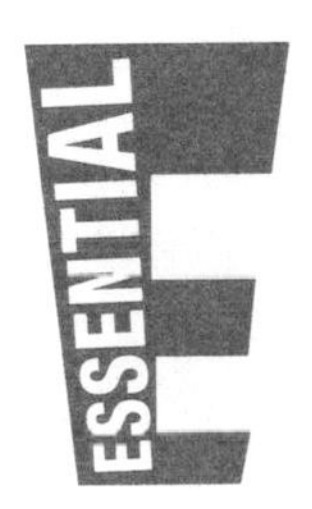

While the term *diabetic* is a useful adjective for describing things and conditions related to diabetes—diabetic supplies, diabetic kidney disease, etc.—many people with the disease bristle at being labeled "a diabetic." People with diabetes should not have to be defined by the disease, nor marginalized because of it.

Pancreatic Tissues

In the pancreas, specialized cells known as *exocrine tissue* secrete digestive enzymes into a network of ducts that join the main pancreatic duct and end up in the duodenum, where they are key in processing carbohydrates, proteins, and other nutrients.

The endocrine tissues of the pancreas contain cell clusters known as *islets of Langerhans*, named after Dr. Paul Langerhans, who first described them in medical literature. Islets (pronounced EYE-lets) are constructed of three cell types:

- **Alpha cells** manufacture and release glucagon, a hormone that raises blood glucose levels.
- **Beta cells** monitor blood sugar levels and produce glucose-lowering insulin in response.
- **Delta cells** produce the hormone somatostatin, which researchers believe is responsible for directing the action of both the beta and alpha cells.

Another Key Player: The Liver

Located toward the front of the abdomen and above the stomach, the liver is the center of glucose storage. This important organ converts glucose—the fuel that the cells of the human body require for energy—into its principal storage form, *glycogen*. Glycogen is warehoused in muscle and in the liver itself, where it can later be converted back to glucose for energy with the help of the hormones epinephrine (secreted by the adrenal glands) and glucagon (from the pancreas).

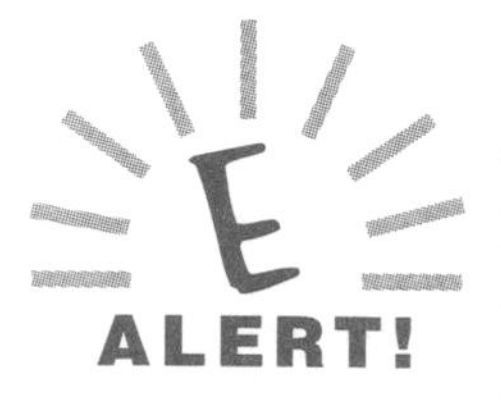

People with type 1 diabetes should always have an emergency glucagon injection kit on hand. Glucagon is a hormone that prompts the liver to release glycogen and convert it into glucose. It is used to treat a severe hypoglycemic episode (severe low blood sugar) in type 1 or type 2 diabetes.

Together, the liver and pancreas preserve a delicate balance of blood glucose and insulin, produced in sufficient amounts to both fuel cells and maintain glycogen storage.

Insulin and Blood Sugar

While the liver is one source of glucose, most glucose the body uses is manufactured from food, primarily carbohydrates. Cells then metabolize, or convert, blood glucose for energy. And insulin is the hormone that makes it all happen.

To visualize the role of insulin in the body and in diabetes, think of a flattened basketball. The ball needs air (or glucose) to supply the necessary energy to bounce. To fill a basketball, you insert an inflating needle into the ball valve to open it, then pump air through it into the ball. Likewise, when a cell needs energy, insulin binds to an insulin receptor, or cell gateway, to "open" the cell and let glucose in for processing.

You can blow pounds and pounds of compressed air at the ball valve, but without a needle to open it, the air will not enter. The same applies to your cells. Without insulin to bind to the receptors and open the cell for glucose, the glucose cannot enter. Instead, it builds up to damaging and toxic levels in the bloodstream.

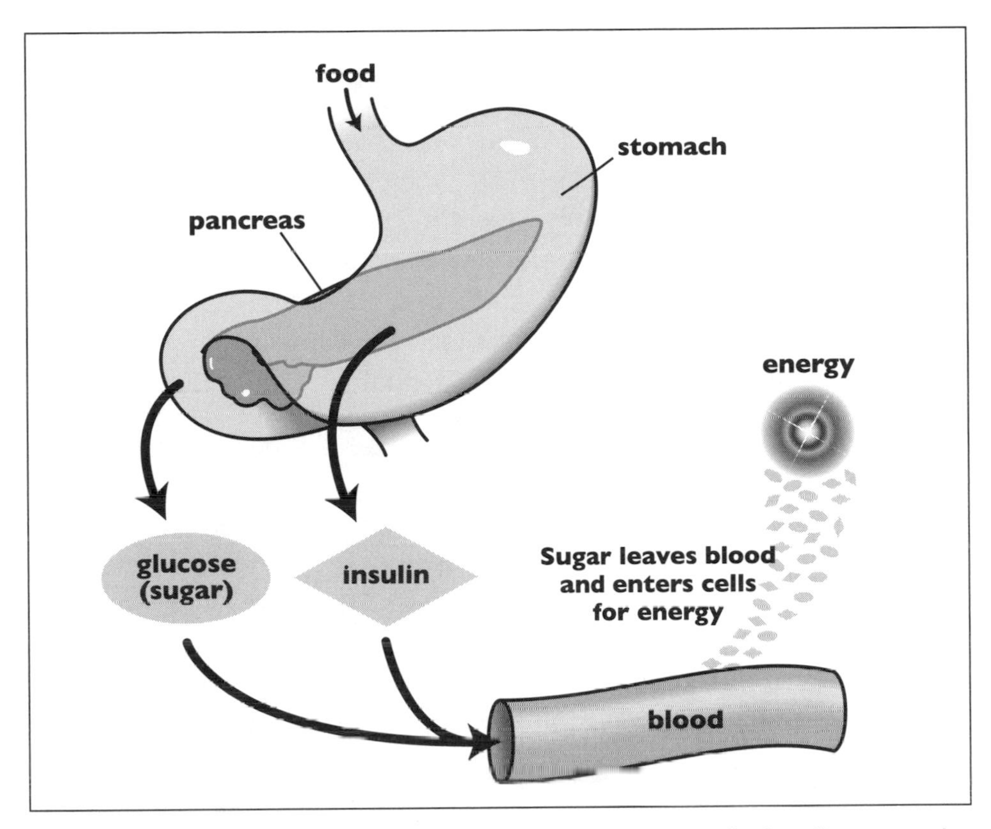

▲ How it works: the pancreas, glucose, and insulin. Normally, insulin enters the bloodstream to regulate the levels of glucose.

What Goes Wrong in Diabetes

In people with type 1 diabetes, the inflating needle is missing (no insulin production), or there are only one or two needles to fit an entire court full of basketballs (insufficient insulin production). This happens when the islets (specifically the insulin-producing beta cells) of the pancreas are destroyed. In people with type 2 diabetes, the inflating needle is the wrong size or shape for the valve (or, in rarer circumstances, the valve itself is too small or missing).

This latter phenomenon, where there's plenty of insulin but the body isn't using it properly, is known as *insulin resistance*. It also occurs in gestational diabetes mellitus (GDM), a type of diabetes that first starts in pregnancy. In some cases, people with type 2 diabetes go on to develop a certain amount of beta cell death and insulin insufficiency as well. Gestational diabetes usually resolves itself after childbirth, although women who develop GDM have a higher risk for developing the permanent insulin resistance of type 2 diabetes later in life.

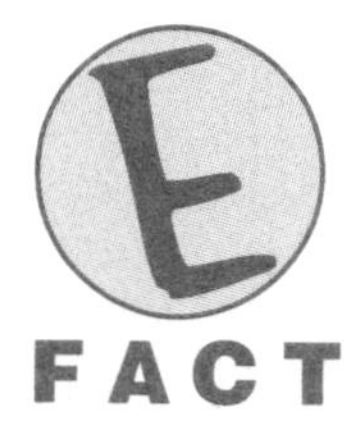

FACT

Although the name is almost the same, diabetes insipidus (also known as *water diabetes*) is a condition completely different in cause and treatment than diabetes mellitus. Diabetes insipidus is characterized by a problem with the kidneys that impedes their ability to concentrate urine adequately, usually due to a deficiency in antidiuretic hormone (ADH).

The human body needs glucose to function, but too much glucose circulating in the bloodstream has the potential to be toxic, a problem known as *glucotoxicity*. When insulin isn't available, blood glucose levels rise higher and higher in the bloodstream. Fatigue, excessive thirst, increased urination, and flulike symptoms such as nausea and vomiting may appear. A severe rise in blood sugar can result in diabetic ketoacidosis (DKA) or hyperglycemic hyperosmolar nonketotic coma (HHNC), sometimes called diabetic coma—both are life-threatening medical emergencies.

A timely diagnosis and immediate treatment are important in preventing DKA, HHNC, and other complications. Long-term, elevated blood sugars can damage virtually all the systems of the body. Blood vessel damage can result in cardiovascular disease, neuropathy (nerve damage), retinopathy (retinal eye disease), nephropathy (kidney disease), and more. To learn more about preventing complications, see Chapter 15.

Managing Diabetes: A Balancing Act

While chronically high glucose levels are the hallmark symptom of diabetes, blood sugars that dip too low are also a hazard of the disease.

Hypoglycemia, or low blood sugar levels, is dangerous because the central nervous system requires glucose to function properly. The most common triggers for a "hypo" are:

- An imbalance of food and insulin, such as when too much insulin is administered for the amount of carbohydrates eaten.
- Exercise without sufficient carb intake.
- Excess alcohol intake.

Some people also experience nighttime dips in blood glucose levels as their liver shuts down glucose production during sleep.

Controlling Blood Glucose

The ultimate goal of management of any type of diabetes mellitus is to bring blood glucose to a level that is as close to normal as possible as consistently as possible. The American Diabetes Association (ADA) suggests people with diabetes try to achieve blood glucose levels of 80 to 120 mg/dl (milligrams per deciliter) or 4.4 to 6.7 mmol/l (millimoles per liter) before meals, and 100 to 140 mg/dl or 5.6 to 7.8 mmol/l at bedtime.

It's important to remember, however, that each patient has unique glucose goals. Those who are particularly susceptible to episodes of hypoglycemia may have a slightly higher baseline goal than those who aren't, while women who are trying to bring their glucose levels down as part of a preconception plan for pregnancy may have a lower baseline for tighter control. Your doctor will work with you to figure out what goals are right for your medical history and lifestyle.

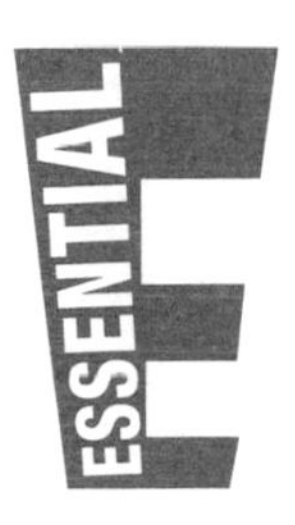

A normal, nonfasting blood glucose reading is between 60 and 140 mg/dl (or 3.3 to 7.8 mmol/l). A casual plasma glucose reading of 200 mg/dl (11.1 mmol/l) or higher, a fasting plasma glucose reading of 126 mg/dl (7.0 mmol/l) or higher, or an oral glucose tolerance test with a two-hour postload value of 200 mg/dl (11.1 mmol/l) or higher are high readings that may indicate diabetes.

Treatment Tools

How do you bring blood sugars down to a controlled range? Each person will have his or her own unique treatment plan, but the main tools at your disposal are diet, exercise, and medication. People with type 1 diabetes require insulin therapy. Those with type 2 diabetes can sometimes control their disease with a combination of dietary regulation and exercise, while others may require some oral medication and/or insulin. No matter what your type of diabetes, proper nutrition and exercise should be a cornerstone of both disease management and healthy living.

The Name Game

Diabetes is the Greek word for "siphon" (since people with uncontrolled diabetes tend to urinate copiously). *Mellitus* is Latin for "honey" or "sweet," a name added when physicians discovered that the urine from people with diabetes is sweet with glucose.

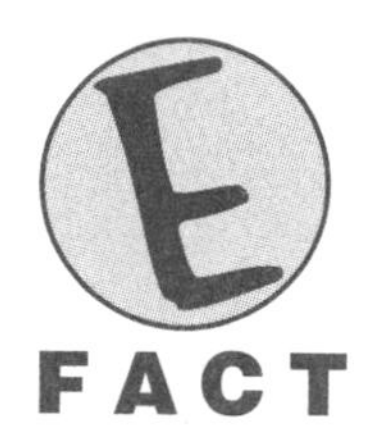
FACT

Long before the advent of diagnostic urine testing in the nineteenth century, one of the earliest ways physicians learned to make a diagnosis of diabetes was to taste a patient's urine.

As researchers began to understand diabetes more, different subtypes of the disease were classified. Type 1 diabetes was once routinely called insulin-dependent diabetes mellitus (or IDDM), and type 2 diabetes was called non-insulin-dependent diabetes mellitus (NIDDM). The problem with this classification scheme was that it defined diabetes not by the cause of the disease, but by its treatment—specifically whether or not a patient required insulin injections. This was often confusing because so-called non-insulin-dependent (type 2) patients do frequently require insulin therapy.

Types and Subtypes of Diabetes

Classification	Includes these clinical subtypes
Type 1	Type 1A LADA* Idiopathic type 1B
Type 2	N/A
Gestational	N/A
Other types, caused by the following:	Genetic beta cell defects (like MODY) Genetic insulin action defects Other genetic syndromes Diseases of or injury to the pancreas Other endocrine disorders Drugs or toxins

For more information on particular types and subtypes of diabetes, read Chapters 2 and 3.

*Not yet officially recognized by the American Diabetes Association.

Also confusing was the system of calling type 1 diabetes "juvenile diabetes" and type 2 diabetes "adult-onset diabetes." While most cases of type 1 diabetes are diagnosed in childhood and adolescence, adults of any age, from twenty-something to the elderly, can develop the disease. And in recent years, type 2 diabetes has begun to appear in younger adults and children as obesity rates soar in the United States. In short, there are no age limits to either type of diabetes.

In the late 1990s, both the American Diabetes Association and the World Health Organization recommended using type 1 diabetes and type 2 diabetes as the clinical standard to explain these very complex, similar yet completely different diseases. However, you may come across a few physicians, and many laypeople, who still use the old monikers.

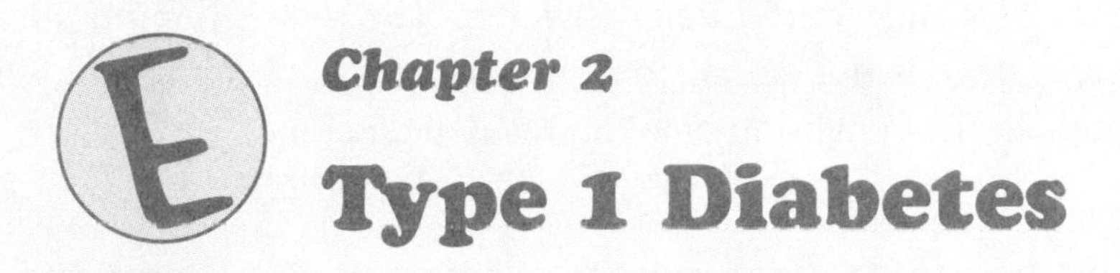

Chapter 2

Type 1 Diabetes

Type 1 diabetes, sometimes called juvenile diabetes, childhood diabetes, or insulin-dependent diabetes mellitus (IDDM), occurs when 90 percent or more of pancreatic beta cells have been destroyed, usually by an autoimmune process that impels the body to attack itself. Consequently, the body produces little to no insulin. Without insulin to assist in processing the glucose, blood sugars rise to damaging and potentially fatal levels.

Type 1A, or Autoimmune, Diabetes

Although there are several different subtypes of type 1 diabetes, the most common form of type 1 diabetes is an autoimmune disease, or an attack from within. For some reason, the T lymphocytes (T cells) don't recognize the beta cells of the pancreas as part of the body, and instead attack them as if they were foreign invaders. The trigger behind this autoimmune siege is not completely understood. Current research points to a combination of environmental and genetic factors.

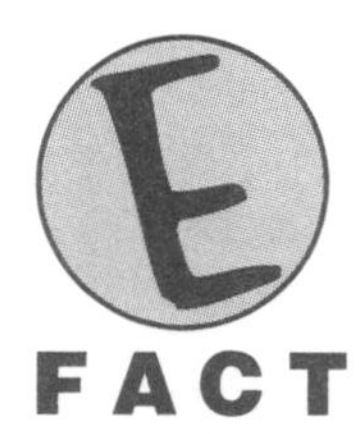

FACT

Certain diseases that damage the pancreas (such as hemochromatosis, cystic fibrosis, and pancreatitis) may cause beta cell destruction that can eventually lead to diabetes and insulin dependence. Some endocrine disorders, including Cushing's syndrome and acromegaly, cause hormone imbalances that influence the way insulin is produced and processed by the body, subsequently leading to diabetes.

Signs of Self-Destruction

An antibody is a protein that works along with T cells and other immune system components to destroy a specific foreign presence in the body, such as bacteria or viruses. An autoantibody is an antibody gone haywire—a substance that attacks cells in the body that it is supposed to protect.

Up to 90 percent of individuals with type 1 diabetes test positive for the presence of islet cell antibodies (ICA), insulin autoantibodies (IAA), and/or autoantibodies to glutamic acid decarboxylase (a beta cell protein known as GAD). These autoantibodies attack the insulin-producing beta cells. A positive islet cell antibody test can actually detect the autoimmune processes that attack the beta cells of the pancreas before clinical symptoms of hyperglycemia (high blood glucose levels) actually occur. When type 1 diabetes is known to be caused by an autoimmune process, it is referred to as *type 1A* diabetes. Immune-mediated type 1 diabetes also puts you at a higher risk for developing other autoimmune disorders, such as celiac disease, thyroid disease, myasthenia gravis, and others.

Latent Autoimmune Diabetes of Adulthood

Yet another subcategory of type 1A diabetes, latent autoimmune diabetes of adulthood (LADA), occurs in approximately 10 percent of all cases of diabetes of adults over age thirty. This immune-mediated form of diabetes is sometimes referred to as late-onset autoimmune diabetes of adulthood, slow-onset type 1, or type 1.5 diabetes. Basically, individuals with LADA experience a slower and longer process of beta cell destruction than those with type 1A diabetes.

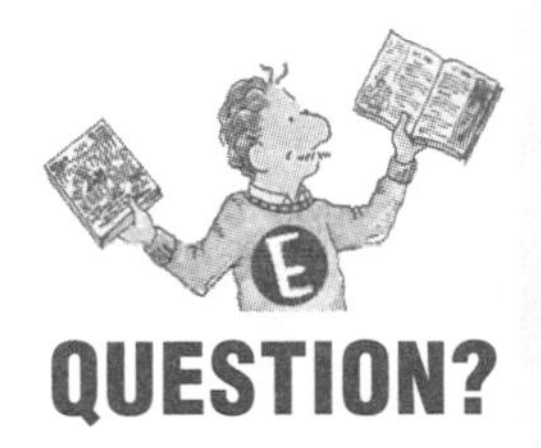

I'm thirty-five, and my doctor just told me I have type 1 diabetes. Don't only kids get that?
The autoimmune processes that cause beta cell destruction may happen very quickly or it may take decades. LADA can be distinguished from type 2 diabetes through blood tests for autoimmune antibodies and c-peptide, a protein that is a by-product of insulin production.

Type 1B, or Idiopathic, Diabetes

Type 1B diabetes is also referred to as *idiopathic diabetes*, or diabetes of unknown origin. This form of type 1 diabetes is not autoimmune in nature, and tests for islet cell antibodies will come up negative. People with type 1B have an insulin deficiency and can experience ketoacidosis (a high blood sugar emergency), but their need for insulin injections typically waxes and wanes over time. Patients of African, Hispanic, or Asian descent are more likely to develop type 1B diabetes.

Genetics and Heredity

Exactly what sets off the complex mechanisms behind beta cell destruction and eventual insulin dependence is not completely understood, but researchers believe that it is likely a genetic predisposition to the disease activated by an environmental trigger.

Genetic Markers

Human leukocyte antigens (HLA) are a set of surface blood proteins that help to control immune function. Two specific HLA markers—HLA-DR and HLA-DQ—help the immune system identify foreign invaders and have been specifically linked with type 1A diabetes.

But while everyone with type 1 diabetes is thought to have one of these genetic markers, not everyone with a marker goes on to develop diabetes. For this reason, genetic testing can be helpful in identifying the possibility of diabetes but not in determining with certainty that it will occur.

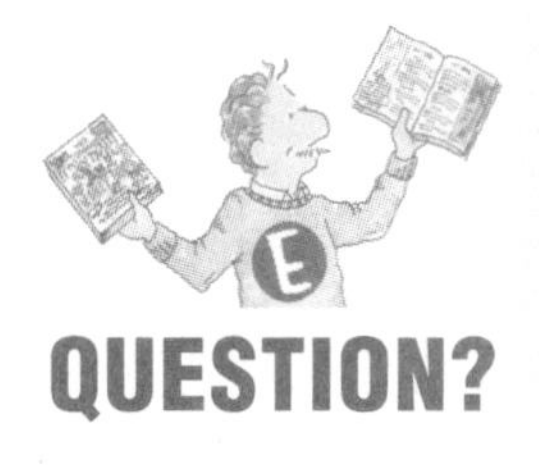

QUESTION?

How do I know if I have type 1A or type 1B diabetes?
The issue is largely an academic one. The expense and scarcity of autoantibody tests at this point in time makes them impractical for routine use, and knowing your type probably won't have any real bearing on the course of treatment. The overall approach to disease management is the same, even though type 1B individuals may have some periods of insulin independence.

In addition to statistical uncertainty, it is also cost-prohibitive to use genetic testing to screen for type 1 diabetes, and because there are no known methods of delaying or preventing the disease if a genetic tendency is revealed, the test serves no practical purpose. In their 2003 Clinical Practice Recommendation, the American Diabetes Association recommends against routine genetic and autoantibody screening (i.e., ICA, IAA, GAD) for type 1 diabetes outside of a clinical trial setting. However, in circumstances where it is unclear if a patient is type 1 or type 2 and early diagnosis may provide a way to preserve some degree of islet cell function, testing may be appropriate.

Family History

Heredity is a relatively small piece of the puzzle in predicting type 1 diabetes. Statistically, people with an immediate family member who has type 1 diabetes are fifteen times more likely than the general population to develop the disease. Yet only 10 percent of people with type 1 have a first-degree relative with the disease.

Having a parent with type 1 places you at an approximate 5 percent risk of developing the disease (2 to 3 percent for the mother and about 6 percent for the father). If you have a sibling with the disease, your risk is an estimated 6 percent.

Looking at cases of type 1 in identical twin studies puts the role of heredity in an even better perspective. In cases where one identical twin develops type 1 diabetes, an estimated 30 to 70 percent of their twin siblings will develop it. In other words, having a carbon copy gene set of someone with diabetes isn't a guarantee that the disease will occur. Something in the environment must flip the switch.

Ethnicity

U.S. epidemiological studies have found that Caucasians have a higher incidence of type 1 diabetes than Hispanics and African-Americans. Interestingly, geography also seems to play a part in the rates of type 1 diabetes among certain populations. For example, Finland and Sardinia (Italy) have the highest incidence of type 1 diabetes worldwide, while Asian countries like Japan and China have extremely low rates of the disease.

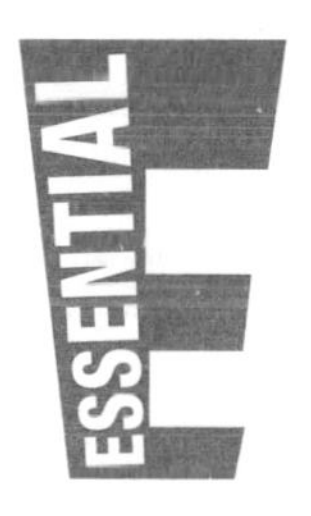

A good way to remember the core difference between type 1 and type 2 diabetes is in terms of insulin processing. People with type 1 diabetes are insulin *deficient*, meaning their pancreas is producing little to no insulin. In contrast, most people with type 2 diabetes initially generate enough insulin, but because they are insulin *resistant*, their bodies can't use it to process blood glucose.

Environmental Triggers

What exactly triggers the autoimmune system to self-destruct is not clear, but studies have implicated several viable theories. Environmental toxins, a virus, or a medication may be the final physiological straw for someone genetically predisposed to the disease.

As of early 2003, clinical studies had implicated fourteen different viruses in beta cell damage and the development of type 1 diabetes, including adenovirus, coxsackie B virus, mumps virus, enteroviruses, rubella virus, cytomegalovirus, and Epstein-Barr virus. It's important to remember, however, that developing one of these viruses does not guarantee you will develop type 1 diabetes; specific genetic programming for the disease must also be present.

Cow's Milk

Exposure to cow's milk and cow's milk–based formula before one year of age has been associated with the development of type 1 diabetes in some studies, although other research has found no link. Study results are also mixed on the role of dietary proteins and their association with the development of autoimmunity and type 1 diabetes in both animal and human trials. In late 2002, the Juvenile Diabetes Research Foundation, the National Institutes of Health, and several other governmental and advocacy organizations announced a large-scale, multinational study called TRIGR (Trial to Reduce Insulin-Dependent Diabetes in the Genetically at Risk). TRIGR will be the first large-scale, long-term study to assess the relationship of infant formula consumption in relation to the likelihood of developing type 1 diabetes in infants considered genetically at risk for developing the disease. The two-year study will involve 6,000 families in fourteen countries, and will hopefully determine with certainty the association, if any, between type 1 diabetes and milk proteins.

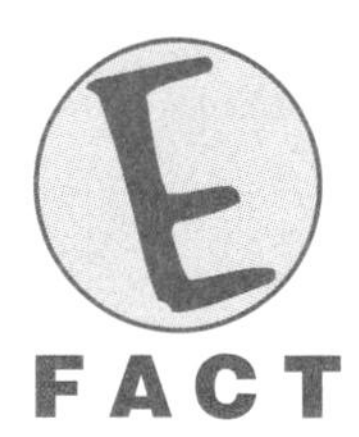

FACT

Clinical research has found that babies who breastfeed at least three months have a lower incidence of type 1 diabetes, and may be less likely to become obese as adults.

Other Causes of Beta Cell Destruction

Certain toxins, drugs, genetic defects, and diseases of the pancreas can also cause beta cell destruction, leading to diabetes mellitus.

The occurrence of diabetes in this category is relatively rare—an estimated 1 to 5 percent of all diagnosed cases of diabetes according to the U.S. Centers for Disease Control (CDC) and the National Institutes of Health (NIH). As such, their causes and specific treatments are not covered in this book.

Signs and Symptoms

Physical signs of type 1 diabetes usually appear rapidly as uncontrolled high blood glucose, or hyperglycemia, reaches crisis levels. Symptoms include the following:

- Excessive thirst
- Frequent urination
- Extreme hunger
- Unexplained weight loss
- Fatigue, or a feeling of being "run down" and tired
- Rapid breathing
- Blurred vision
- Dry, itchy skin
- Headaches
- Tingling or burning pain in the feet, legs, hands, or other parts of the body
- High blood pressure
- Mood swings, irritability, and depression
- Frequent or recurring infections, such as urinary tract infections, yeast infections, and skin infections
- Slow healing of cuts and bruises

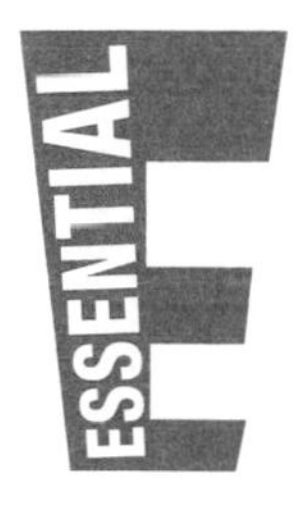

A blood plasma glucose test, either casual (any time of day) or fasting (no food or drink eight hours prior), is used to diagnose type 1 diabetes. If the first test indicates diabetes, a second test on a subsequent day is required to confirm the diagnosis. Turn to Chapter 6 to read about these tests in detail.

Diabetic Ketoacidosis (DKA)

When blood glucose levels are extremely high (above 250 mg/dl or 13.9 mmol/l), signs of DKA may also start to appear. Ketoacidosis is life-threatening and requires immediate medical attention. Symptoms of DKA include the following:

- Lethargy
- Nausea and vomiting
- Abdominal pain
- Fruity breath odor
- Rapid breathing
- Dehydration
- Loss of consciousness

DKA is also diagnosed by the presence of ketones in the urine. (For more on urine testing for ketones, see Chapter 6.)

Hyperglycemic Hyperosmolar Nonketotic Coma (HHNC)

Individuals with type 1 diabetes can also develop a condition known as hyperglycemic hyperosmolar nonketotic coma (HHNC), which is characterized by many of the same symptoms as DKA, and occurs when blood sugar levels are in excess of 600 mg/dl (33.3 mmol/l). HHNS (Hyperglycemic Hyperosmolar Nonketotic Syndrome) is rare in type 1 diabetes, and occurs more frequently in people with type 2 diabetes.

Insulin Is Not a Cure

Subcutaneous injections of insulin are the frontline treatment for type 1 diabetes. However, it's important to realize that insulin is not a cure for diabetes, nor can insulin treatment erase the potential for complications and increased risk for other autoimmune disorders that accompany the disease. The only current "cure" for the disease is the transplantation of a healthy, functioning pancreas or of insulin-producing beta cells, and even that procedure is not without its own set of risks and potential problems (see Chapter 22).

The finely tuned internal biological mechanisms that dispense just the right amount of insulin in response to blood glucose levels are absent in type 1 diabetes patients. While injected exogenous insulin (insulin produced outside of the body) can bring blood glucose levels down to a safe level, it is a far from perfect system. The type and amount of insulin and the timing and location of injections are just a few of the many factors that influence how well the treatment works. The dose of insulin must adequately cover the amount of carbohydrates that will be eaten and the corresponding rise in blood sugar levels. Too much insulin, and hypoglycemia (or low blood glucose) results. Too little, and blood sugars rise too high. Precision is important, yet can be elusive.

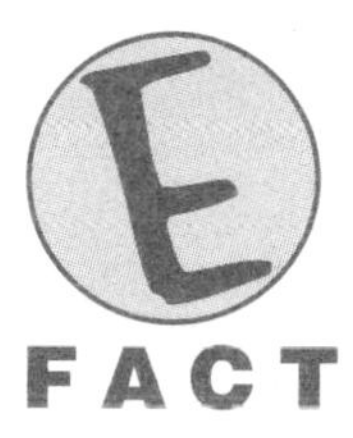

Children and adults diagnosed with type 1 diabetes sometimes experience a period of remission known as the "honeymoon period," which usually occurs shortly after diagnosis as blood glucose levels are brought under control. During a "honeymoon," the remaining islets are functioning sufficiently and the need for insulin injections is greatly reduced or sometimes even eliminated completely.

Vigilant attention to diet, a good understanding of how changes in carb intake affect insulin dose, and basic math skills are essential to proper treatment; yet, even with these, insulin can often be a crap shoot. Circumstances such as emotional stress, use of other medications, and even something as seemingly simple as the common cold can result in skyrocketing blood glucose levels and a potential diabetic emergency. For more on insulin treatment, see Chapter 8.

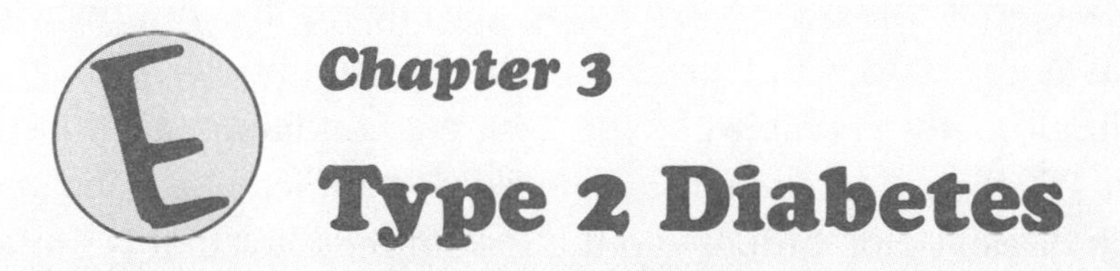

Chapter 3

Type 2 Diabetes

Type 2 diabetes, the most common type of diabetes, is also one of the most prevalent chronic diseases around. Worldwide, more than 150 million people suffer from the disease; the International Diabetes Federation projects that this population will double globally by the year 2025. While weight is a major risk factor for type 2 diabetes, ethnic background, family history, and certain components of your health profile also play an important role.

Insulin Resistance and Type 2

Like type 1 diabetes, type 2 diabetes is a metabolic disorder in which blood glucose rises because it isn't being effectively balanced and metabolized into cell energy by insulin. The similarities in physiology between the two diseases end there, however.

Type 2 diabetes is not caused by the absence of the hormone insulin, as is the case with type 1, but rather by the body's inability to use insulin properly. People with type 2 have a condition called insulin resistance. They can produce insulin, usually in sufficient amounts at first, but it doesn't bind properly to the insulin receptor that is the gateway to cells in muscle, fat, and liver tissue, and they are therefore resistant to its effects. In other words, it's like trying to fit a square peg (insulin) into a round hole (insulin receptor). As a result, glucose doesn't enter the cells and instead builds up in the bloodstream, resulting in high blood sugar levels.

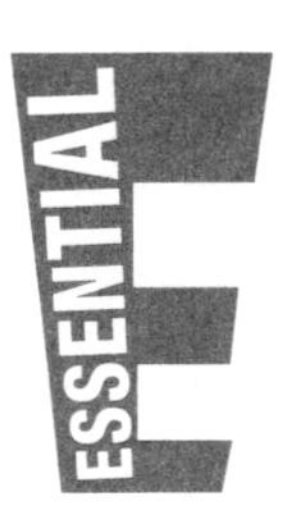

The causes of type 2 diabetes are complex and not completely understood, although research is uncovering new clues at a rapid pace. Animal studies have associated certain genetic markers with the development of the disease, and its relationship with obesity has become clearer in recent years.

The second condition that sets the stage for type 2 diabetes is insulin deficiency—the pancreas also has difficulty producing sufficient amounts of insulin to process the rising blood glucose levels. Eventually it does not have sufficient amounts to overcome the deficit. The toxic effects of long-term high glucose levels on the insulin-producing beta cells on the pancreas (glucotoxicity) can make insulin deficiency worse.

Some people with type 2 are highly insulin resistant with a small amount of related insulin deficiency. Others are primarily insulin deficient and just slightly insulin resistant.

Prediabetes

Type 2 diabetes does not strike without warning. Prediabetes, also known as impaired glucose tolerance (IGT) or impaired fasting glucose (IFG), precedes the condition by months, years, and sometimes even decades.

As the name suggests, prediabetes is defined by blood glucose levels that are higher than normal, but not high enough to indicate diabetes. The actual clinical criterion for a diagnosis of prediabetes is blood glucose level of 110 to 125 mg/dl (6.1 to 6.9 mmol/l), as determined by a fasting blood glucose test, or a two-hour glucose level rising to 140 to 199 mg/dl (7.8 to 11.0 mmol/l). Prediabetes is a signal that without some healthy lifestyle changes, you are most certainly on the path to full-fledged type 2 diabetes. And having prediabetes is a danger in itself. It increases the likelihood of stroke and heart disease by 50 percent, and may also be associated with an increased risk of colon cancer.

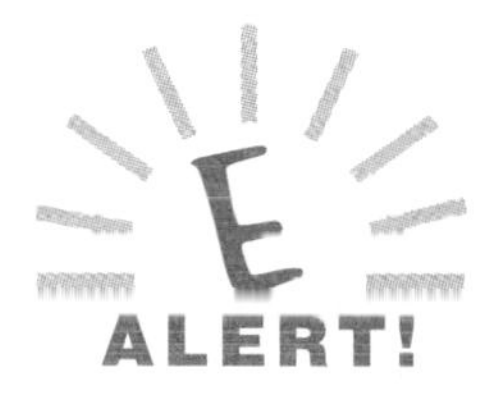

One of the reasons for the boom in type 2 diabetes is the widening of waistbands and the trend toward a more sedentary lifestyle in the United States and other developed countries. In America, the shift has been dramatic; in the 1990s alone, obesity increased by 61 percent and diagnosed diabetes by 49 percent.

Am I at Risk?

Known risk factors for both prediabetes and type 2 diabetes include:

- Being overweight or obese.
- Family history of diabetes.
- Low HDL cholesterol (less than 35 mg/dl, or 1.9 mmol/l) and high triglycerides (higher than 250 mg/dl).
- High blood pressure (consistent reading of 140/90 mmHg or higher).
- History of gestational diabetes.
- Giving birth to a baby weighing more than 9 pounds.
- Belonging to one of the following minority groups: African-Americans, Native American Indians, Hispanic Americans/Latinos, and Asian American/Pacific Islanders.

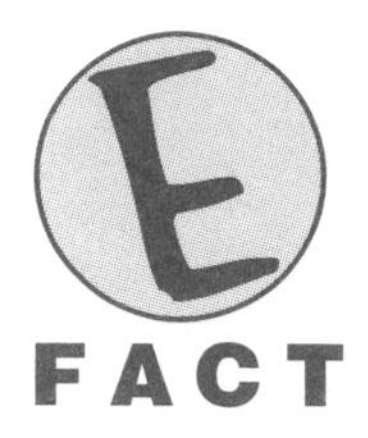

According to the U.S. Department of Health and Human Services, an estimated 16 million Americans have prediabetes—almost as many as are diagnosed with type 2 itself. Many are unaware of their condition. Worse, almost 6 million Americans who have full-blown diabetes remain undiagnosed.

Progression to Type 2 Diabetes

The pancreas of a person with type 2 diabetes generates insulin, but the body is unable to process it in sufficient amounts to control blood sugar levels. In some cases this is due to the chemical makeup of the insulin itself, but most of the time it is connected to how the body's cells—specifically the insulin receptors that attract and process the hormone—recognize and use insulin. As blood glucose levels rise, the pancreas pumps out more and more insulin to try to compensate. This may bring down blood sugar levels to a degree, but also results in high levels of circulating insulin, a condition known as hyperinsulinemia. At a certain threshold, the weakened pancreas cannot produce enough insulin; in some cases insulin secretion is actually reduced by the toxicity of high glucose levels to pancreatic beta cells. At this point, type 2 diabetes results.

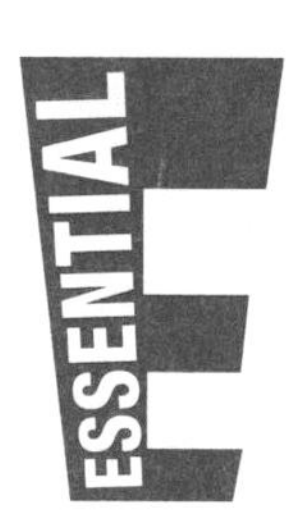

While most people with type 2 diabetes have some degree of insulin resistance, not everyone with insulin resistance has type 2 diabetes. Metabolic syndrome X is a constellation of symptoms—insulin resistance, low HDL and high LDL and triglycerides, excess abdominal fat, and high blood pressure—that puts you at risk for heart disease.

Risk Factors

The biggest indicator for your risk of type 2 diabetes is the diagnosed presence of prediabetes. But since the vast majority of people with prediabetes remain undiagnosed, assessing the presence of the other common risk factors for type 2 diabetes is important.

Age and Ethnicity

According to the American Diabetes Association, over half of all cases of type 2 occur in people over age fifty-five, and close to 7 million Americans age sixty-five and older suffer from the disease. Individuals over age forty-five should be tested for diabetes, and retested every three years thereafter if the initial test is normal.

Certain ethnic groups and minorities have an increased risk of developing type 2 diabetes. These include:

- African-Americans
- Asian-Americans
- Hispanics
- Pacific Islanders
- Native Americans

Family History

Heredity plays a large part in the development of type 2 diabetes. If you have a first-degree relative with type 2 diabetes, your chances of developing the disease double. And there is a concordance rate of up to 90 percent among identical twins with type 2, meaning that in up to 90 percent of cases where one twin has the disease, the other one develops it as well.

The good news for those with diabetes in their family tree is that large-scale studies such as the Diabetes Prevention Program (DPP) have proved that prevention is often possible through diet, exercise, and other moderate lifestyle changes. See Chapter 22 for more on the DPP and what it means to you if you have type 2 diabetes.

Hypertension and Cholesterol Levels

Hypertension, or blood pressure higher than 140/90mmHg, is both a possible complication of type 2 diabetes and a risk factor for the development of the disease. A large-scale study of over 12,000 patients published in the *New England Journal of Medicine* in 2000 found that people with diagnosed hypertension were 2.5 times more likely to develop type 2 diabetes than those with normal blood pressure levels. In addition, that study and others have shown a correlation between beta-blockers, a medication used to treat high blood pressure, and an increased risk of type 2.

Triglyceride levels over 250 mg/dl and levels of HDL (or "good cholesterol") under 35 mg/dl put you at an increased risk for type 2 diabetes. HDL acts as a lubricant for the circulatory system, moving the other lipids (triglycerides and LDL cholesterol) through the blood vessels and into the liver for metabolism. It helps to prevent the buildup of fatty plaque that can otherwise clog the arteries, resulting in atherosclerosis and consequently high blood pressure. Elevated triglycerides are associated with an increased risk of heart disease as well.

Gestational Diabetes and Perinatal Risk Factors

Women who had gestational diabetes mellitus (GDM) during their pregnancy are at an increased risk of developing type 2 diabetes; statistically, between 20 and 50 percent of women with a history of GDM will go on to develop type 2 within five to ten years after giving birth. Giving birth to a baby weighing over 9 pounds is also considered a risk factor for later development of type 2.

Studies have also associated a low birth weight (under 2,500 grams, or 5.5 pounds) with a child's increased risk for type 2 later in life, possibly due to poor fetal nutrition. And high birth weights (over 4,000 grams, or 8.8 pounds) have been linked to type 2 in several studies as well, although the evidence is currently mixed on whether this is a reliable marker of type 2 risk.

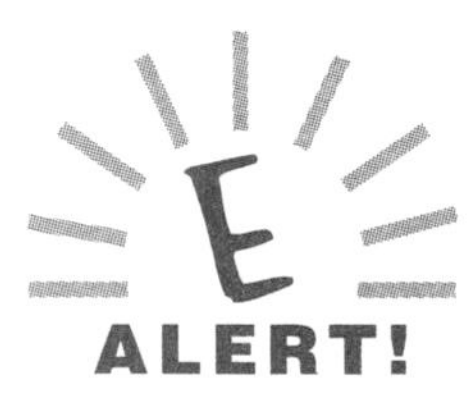

Women who have a history of gestational diabetes should be vigilant about regular testing for diabetes (once every three years if their glucose levels are normal postpartum, annually if they are not). See Chapter 4 for more on gestational diabetes.

Risk Associated with Weight and BMI

The Surgeon General estimates that 61 percent of U.S. adults are overweight, as are 13 percent of children and adolescents. Obesity has been on a steady rise over the past few decades, with nearly one-third of all adults over age twenty classified as obese, according to the 1999–2000 National Health and Nutrition Examination Survey (NHANES).

Being overweight or obese is a primary risk factor for developing prediabetes and type 2 diabetes. The U.S. Department of Health and Human Services (HHS) reports that over 80 percent of people with type 2 diabetes are clinically overweight.

Why Is Weight a Risk Factor?

Too much fat makes it difficult for the body to use its own insulin to process blood glucose and bring it down to normal circulating levels. Why? There are three reasons:

- **Overweight people have fewer available insulin receptors.** When compared to muscle cells, fat cells have fewer insulin receptors, the place where the insulin binds with the cell and "unlocks" it to process glucose into energy.
- **More fat requires more insulin.** The pancreas starts producing larger and larger quantities of insulin in order to "feed" body mass, and consequently insulin resistance turns into a catch-22. Excess blood sugar must be stored as fat, and excess fat promotes further insulin resistance.
- **Fat cells release free fatty acids (FFAs).** Fat cells and tissue, particularly abdominal fat, release free fatty acids, which interfere with glucose metabolism.

Leptin, a hormone in fat cells that helps to metabolize fatty acids, has provided an important clue to the relationship between obesity and type 2 diabetes. Discovered by Rockefeller University researchers in 1995, leptin (after the Greek *leptos*, meaning "thin") also plays a part in sending a satiety—or "all full"—signal to the brain to stop eating when body fat

BMI	19	20	21	22	23	24	25	26	27	28	29	30	31	32	33	34	35	36	37	38	39	40	41	42	43	44	45	46	47	48	49	50	51	52	53	54
Height (inches)	Body weight (pounds)																																			
58	91	96	100	105	110	115	119	124	129	134	138	143	148	153	158	162	167	172	177	181	186	191	196	201	205	210	215	220	224	229	234	239	244	248	253	258
59	94	99	104	109	114	119	124	128	133	138	143	148	153	158	163	168	173	178	183	188	193	198	203	208	212	217	222	227	232	237	242	247	252	257	262	267
60	97	102	107	112	118	123	128	133	138	143	148	153	158	163	168	174	179	184	189	194	199	204	209	215	220	225	230	235	240	245	250	255	261	266	271	276
61	100	106	111	116	122	127	132	137	143	148	153	158	164	169	174	180	185	190	195	201	206	211	217	222	227	232	238	243	248	254	259	264	269	275	280	285
62	104	109	115	120	126	131	136	142	147	153	158	164	169	175	180	186	191	196	202	207	213	218	224	229	235	240	246	251	256	262	267	273	278	284	289	295
63	107	113	118	124	130	135	141	146	152	158	163	169	175	180	186	191	197	203	208	214	220	225	231	237	242	248	254	259	265	270	278	282	287	293	299	304
64	110	116	122	128	134	140	145	151	157	163	169	174	180	186	192	197	204	209	215	221	227	232	238	244	250	256	262	267	273	279	285	291	296	302	308	314
65	114	120	126	132	138	144	150	156	162	168	174	180	186	192	198	204	210	216	222	228	234	240	246	252	258	264	270	276	282	288	294	300	306	312	318	324
66	118	124	130	136	142	148	155	161	167	173	179	186	192	198	204	210	216	223	229	235	241	247	253	260	266	272	278	284	291	297	303	309	315	322	328	334
67	121	127	134	140	146	153	159	166	172	178	185	191	198	204	211	217	223	230	236	242	249	255	261	268	274	280	287	293	299	306	312	319	325	331	338	344
68	125	131	138	144	151	158	164	171	177	184	190	197	203	210	216	223	230	236	243	249	256	262	269	276	282	289	295	302	308	315	322	328	335	341	348	354
69	128	135	142	149	155	162	169	176	182	189	196	203	209	216	223	230	236	243	250	257	263	270	277	284	291	297	304	311	318	324	331	338	345	351	358	365
70	132	139	146	153	160	167	174	181	188	195	202	209	216	222	229	236	243	250	257	264	271	278	285	292	299	306	313	320	327	334	341	348	355	362	369	376
71	136	143	150	157	165	172	179	186	193	200	208	215	222	229	236	243	250	257	265	272	279	286	293	301	308	315	322	329	338	343	351	358	365	372	379	386
72	140	147	154	162	169	177	184	191	199	206	213	221	228	235	242	250	258	265	272	279	287	294	302	309	316	324	331	338	346	353	361	368	375	383	390	397
73	144	151	159	166	174	182	189	197	204	212	219	227	235	242	250	257	265	272	280	288	295	302	310	318	325	333	340	348	355	363	371	378	386	393	401	408
74	148	155	163	171	179	186	194	202	210	218	225	233	241	249	256	264	272	280	287	295	303	311	319	326	334	342	350	358	365	373	381	389	396	404	412	420
75	152	160	168	176	184	192	200	208	216	224	232	240	248	256	264	272	279	287	295	303	311	319	327	335	343	351	359	367	375	383	391	399	407	415	423	431
76	156	164	172	180	189	197	205	213	221	230	238	246	254	263	271	279	287	295	304	312	320	328	336	344	353	361	369	377	385	394	402	410	418	426	435	443
	Normal						Overweight					Obese										Extreme Obesity														

▲ Body mass index (BMI) table

Source: Adapted from *Clinical Guidelines on the Identification, Evaluation, and Treatment of Overweight and Obesity in Adults: The Evidence Report*

increases, and an "empty" signal when body fat is insufficient. It appears that a type of leptin resistance may lead to a situation where fatty acids are deposited instead of metabolized, leading to eventual insulin resistance.

Your BMI

Obesity and body fat are measured by body mass index (BMI)—a number that expresses weight in relationship to height and is a reliable indicator of overall body fat. People with a BMI of 25 to 29.9 are considered overweight; those with a BMI of 30 or over are obese. Extreme obesity is classified as a BMI of 40 or higher.

The NIDDK (National Institute of Diabetes & Digestive & Kidney Diseases) reports that 67 percent of people with type 2 diabetes have a BMI of 27 or higher and 46 percent have a BMI of 30 or higher. You should aim for a BMI of 18.5 to 24.9, which is considered normal.

BMI for children and young adults ages two to twenty is calculated differently. A charting system called BMI-for-age compares each child's weight in relation to other children of the same age and gender on a growth chart in terms of percentiles. For example, a girl in the thirtieth percentile would weigh the same or more than 30 percent of girls the same age.

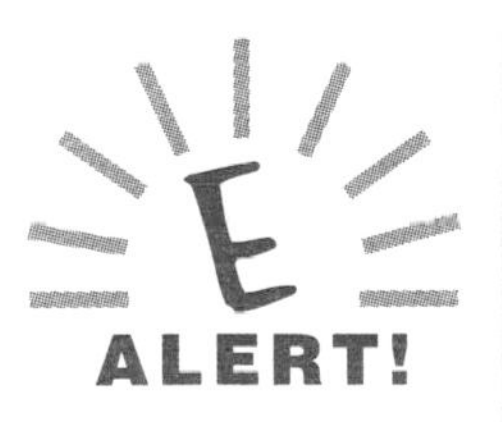

You know smoking is bad for your health, but did you also know it can increase your diabetes risk? Smoking constricts blood vessels, raising blood pressure and increasing the risk of coronary artery disease. It also stimulates the release of catecholamines, which have been shown to promote insulin resistance.

A BMI-for-age that is equal to or over the ninety-fifth percentile is considered overweight, while the eighty-fifth to ninety-fourth percentile is "at risk" for being overweight. Growth charts used for assessing pediatric BMI-for-age are based on National Health and Nutrition Examination Survey (NHANES) data and generated by the U.S. Centers for Disease Control (CDC). The CDC Web site (*www.cdc.gov*) has more information.

Body Shape

Having an apple-shaped body, with excess pounds packed in the midsection rather than the hips, is another hallmark of insulin resistance. In fact, the National Institutes of Health recommends that waist circumference be used as a screening tool for evaluating the risk of heart disease and type 2 diabetes.

Classification of Overweight and Obesity by BMI, Waist Circumference, and Associated Risk of Type 2 Diabetes, Hypertension, and Cardiovascular Disease

		Disease Risk Relative to Normal Weight and Waist Circumference	
	BMI (kg/m^2)	≤102 cm (≤40 in.) for men; ≤88 cm (≤35 in.) for women	>102 cm (>40 in.) for men; >88 cm (>35 in.) for women
Underweight	<18.5	no risk	no risk
Normal	18.5–24.9	no risk	no risk
Overweight	25.0–29.9	increased	high
Obesity	30.0–34.9	high	very high
	35.0–39.9	very high	very high
Extreme Obesity	≥40	extremely high	extremely high

From the National Institutes of Health; National Heart, Lung, and Blood Institute

Another type 2 risk sometimes related to weight is an inactive lifestyle. Exercise, even at a moderate level, reduces blood glucose levels. People who lead sedentary lifestyles, exercising less than three times a week, are more likely to develop type 2 diabetes than those who get up and move on a regular basis.

Signs and Symptoms

Both type 1 and type 2 diabetes exhibit the same basic symptoms of hyperglycemia. Some symptoms, such as tingling or burning in the hands and feet (neuropathy), are the result of long-term uncontrolled blood glucose, and are more common in type 2 patients. It's important to note that not all people with type 2 diabetes will have symptoms, particularly in the early stages of the disease. In fact, up to a third of all Americans with type 2 diabetes are unaware that they have it.

Symptoms of type 2 diabetes may include one or more of the following:

- Thirst and frequent urination
- Dry, itchy skin
- Headache
- Tingling or burning pain in the feet, legs, hands, or other parts of the body
- High blood pressure
- Mood swings (i.e., irritability, depression)
- Fatigue, or a feeling of being "run down" and tired
- Blurred vision
- Extreme hunger
- Unexplained weight loss
- Frequent or recurring infections (e.g., urinary tract infections, yeast infections)
- Slow healing of cuts and bruises

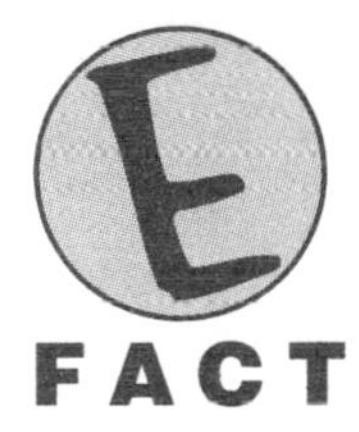

Women of reproductive age who have developed polycystic ovarian syndrome (PCOS) are at an increased risk for type 2 diabetes. PCOS is a hormonal disorder characterized by enlarged ovaries containing fluid-filled cysts. Women with PCOS have irregular menstrual cycles and high circulating levels of male hormones (like testosterone). Insulin resistance and impaired glucose tolerance are manifestations of PCOS.

Hyperglycemic Hyperosmolar Nonketotic Coma

When blood glucose levels exceed 600 mg/dl (33.3 mmol/l), a condition known as hyperglycemic hyperosmolar nonketotic coma (HHNC) may occur. In HHNS, the body becomes severely dehydrated and fluids are depleted from the bloodstream. Older adults tend to develop HHNS more readily, although the condition can occur at any age.

HHNS is life-threatening and requires immediate medical attention. Symptoms of the syndrome include:

- Dehydration
- Excessive thirst
- Nausea and vomiting
- Fever
- Hypotension (low blood pressure that may be signaled by dizziness or faintness)
- Disorientation
- Sudden excessive sleepiness
- Seizures
- Visual disturbances and/or hallucinations
- In extreme cases, coma or hemiplegia (paralysis or weakness on one side of the body)

Hyperinsulinemia

Hyperglycemia is not the only danger in type 2 diabetes. As glucose levels build up in the bloodstream, the pancreas kicks out more and more insulin in an effort to bring them back down. Consistently high levels of circulating insulin is a condition known as *hyperinsulinemia*.

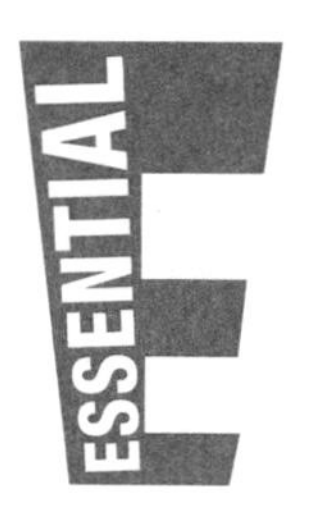

People with type 2 can also develop diabetic ketoacidosis (DKA), but it is not as common as it is in type 1 diabetes, and generally only occurs as a result of a major physical stressor such as a heart attack.

Diagnosing Type 2 Diabetes

A blood plasma glucose test, either casual (any time of day) or fasting (no food or drink eight hours prior), is used to diagnose type 2 diabetes. A normal, nonfasting blood glucose reading is between 60 and 140 mg/dl

(3.3–7.8 mmol/l). A casual plasma glucose reading of 200 mg/dl (11.1 mmol/l) or higher, a fasting plasma glucose reading of 126 mg/dl (7.0 mmol/l) or higher, or an oral glucose tolerance test with a two-hour postload value of 200 mg/dl (11.1 mmol/l) or higher are high readings that may indicate diabetes. For more on diagnosing diabetes, see Chapter 5.

Long-term uncontrolled blood glucose levels can cause major damage to virtually every system in the body, head to toes. If you are experiencing any of the symptoms of diabetes, it's crucial to visit a health care professional as soon as possible for evaluation. If a diagnosis is made, maintaining tight control of your blood glucose levels is the best way to avoid serious complications.

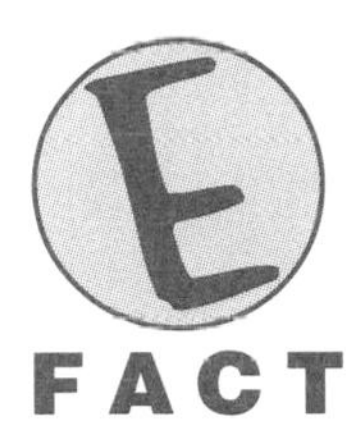

FACT

Maturity-onset diabetes in the young (MODY) is a rare form of diabetes caused by a specific genetic defect of beta cell function. Although MODY is treated like type 2 diabetes, with diet, exercise, and occasionally oral medications, it is a distinctly different class of diabetes.

Not Just for Adults Anymore

Type 2 diabetes, once considered an "adults-only" disease, is appearing in children and teens in epidemic proportions. In 2000, an expert panel of the American Diabetes Association estimated that on average 20 percent of newly diagnosed diabetes in children was type 2, and 85 percent of those children were obese.

This alarming surge in childhood type 2 has been fueled by the fast-food, video-centric culture that is part of today's lifestyle. Children lead a more sedentary lifestyle centered around passive entertainment mediums like television and online gaming; supersized, high-fat, low-fiber convenience food has become a dietary staple in the quest for quick and easy. As a result, an estimated 13 percent of children six to eleven years old and 14 percent of adolescents twelve to nineteen years old in the United States are overweight according to the U.S. Surgeon General. A 2002 study published in the *New England Journal of Medicine* found that impaired glucose tolerance and insulin resistance are highly prevalent in children and adolescents who are obese.

Kids at Risk

The same factors that place adults at great risk for type 2 diabetes apply to children as well. Obesity is far and away the primary threat in this age group.

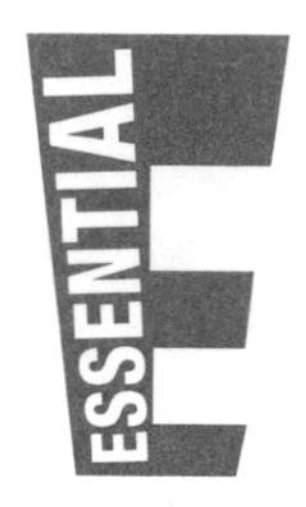

Acanthosis nigricans (darkening of the skin) is present in up to 90 percent of children and adolescents who develop type 2 diabetes. This condition is a clinical sign of insulin resistance and is more common in people with darker skin pigmentation. The dark, velvety patches typically appear in areas where skin folds gather—on the neck, armpits, and groin—and are associated with high levels of circulating insulin (hyperinsulinemia).

Having a family history of type 2 diabetes among first- and second-degree relatives and being of African-American, Native American, Asian, Pacific Island, or Hispanic descent also increase the likelihood that overweight children will develop the disease.

The majority of childhood type 2 cases are diagnosed at puberty or beyond. Puberty itself is the cause of a certain degree of insulin resistance in adolescents, which is thought to be triggered by a natural rise in growth hormone during this time. In children who are already disposed toward the disease, insulin resistance remains even after growth hormone returns to normal levels.

Treating Kids for an Adult Disease

Diagnoses of type 2 in children are sometimes difficult to make, especially in children who are not overtly obese. Many physicians still consider type 2 diabetes an adults-only disease. And it can present the same way as type 1, with DKA or, in extreme cases, HHNS. Often because of the age of the patient, type 1 is initially suspected and the child begins insulin treatment. However, long-term use of insulin after blood sugars have stabilized can contribute to further weight gain, which can worsen the problem.

Children diagnosed with type 2 diabetes can usually be treated through a combination of diet and exercise. Oral medications may be helpful, but clinical data is limited on their long-term effects in children. As of early 2003, metformin was the only oral agent FDA approved for use in pediatric populations (over age ten). However, other oral agents are sometimes prescribed for off-label use in children.

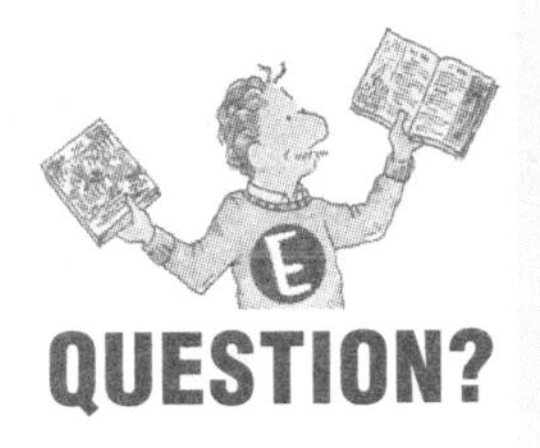

My daughter is overweight, but we have no history of diabetes in our family. Should I really be concerned about her weight?

Yes. Weight problems in childhood can lead to the development of a host of medical problems, like atherosclerosis, hypertension, respiratory infections, sleep apnea, and type 2 diabetes. Talk to her pediatrician about a weight-loss strategy. And remember, diet and exercise should become a family affair to ensure the greatest chance of success for your daughter.

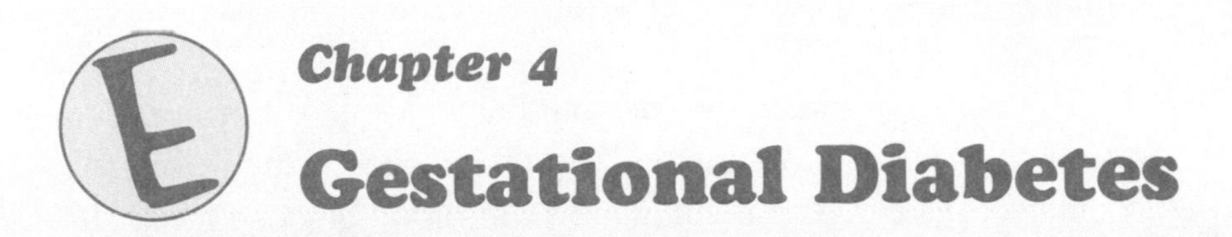

Chapter 4

Gestational Diabetes

Gestational diabetes, also known as gestational diabetes mellitus or GDM, is diabetes that women develop during pregnancy. It occurs in about 200,000 cases, or 7 percent, of U.S. pregnancies annually. Some women with GDM will go on to develop type 2 diabetes later in life; it's been estimated that having GDM in pregnancy increases your type 2 risk by up to 50 percent.

Diabetes, Your Baby, and You

Gestational diabetes is similar to type 2 diabetes in that both are caused by a phenomenon known as *insulin resistance*. People who are insulin resistant can produce insulin, but either their insulin receptors prevent it from binding correctly and allowing glucose to enter the cell, or, less commonly, there is something wrong with the insulin itself that makes it unable to work.

The placenta that is feeding your baby produces hormones, including estrogen, cortisol, and human placental lactogen, which work to counteract insulin. The result is a rise in blood glucose levels. In most pregnant women this rise is inconsequential, but in those who have developed significant insulin resistance, it grows to unmanageable levels and GDM results.

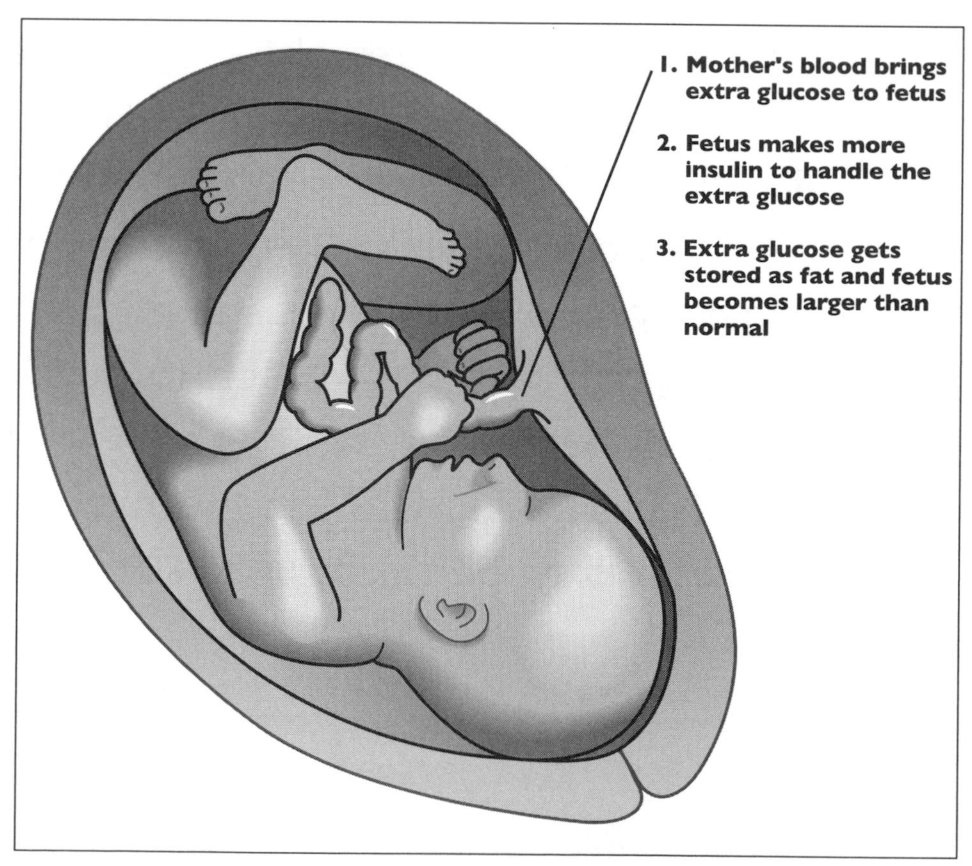

▲ How macrosomia occurs.

A Danger to You and Your Baby

Uncontrolled high blood sugar is damaging to both you and your baby. Over time, it can damage your nervous system, contribute to cardiovascular problems, impair your kidney function, and make you more vulnerable to infection. It can also increase your risk of developing high blood pressure, and possible pre-eclampsia, in pregnancy.

High fasting blood glucose levels have been associated with an increased risk of fetal death in the final eight weeks of pregnancy. GDM also increases your child's risk of developing macrosomia, which can complicate delivery and has the potential to result in a birth injury (such as shoulder dystocia).

And because your diabetes can cause your child's lungs to develop at a slower rate, she is at risk for respiratory distress syndrome, a condition in which inadequate production of surfactant (the substance that enables the alveoli, or air sacs, of the lungs to expand) makes breathing difficult for your baby after she is born.

Who Is at Risk?

Your age, ethnicity, weight, and medical history all factor into your risk for developing gestational diabetes. You are considered at an increased risk for gestational diabetes if any one or more of the following risk factors apply:

- You belong to certain high-risk ethnic groups, including Hispanics, Native Americans, African-Americans, Asian-Americans, and Pacific Islanders.
- You're overweight (as defined by a body mass index, or BMI, of 25 or higher).
- You have a first-degree relative with diabetes.
- You're over age twenty-five.
- You have a history of GDM.
- You have a history of impaired glucose tolerance.
- You have had a baby weighing 9 pounds or more in a past pregnancy.

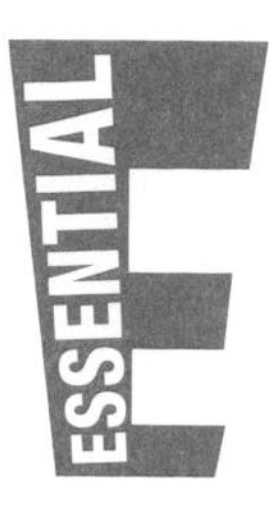

The National Institutes of Health recommends that women with two or more risk factors should be tested as soon as they become pregnant, and again between twenty-four and twenty-eight weeks of pregnancy. Women with a single risk factor can wait until the twenty-fourth week to be tested.

GDM Diagnosis

The first sign that you've developed GDM may be glycosuria, or the sudden appearance of glucose in your urine. Virtually every pregnant woman spills a small amount of glucose into her urine, but if your doctor detects significant glycosuria during a routine urine test, she may order a plasma glucose test to measure the level of glucose in your blood. A level of 126 mg/dl (7.0 mmol/l) or higher if you had been fasting at the time of the blood test, or 200 mg/dl (11.1 mmol/l) or higher if you were not, points to hyperglycemia (high blood sugar) and gestational diabetes. However, you must have your blood retested on a subsequent day to confirm that diagnosis.

Without any obvious signs or symptoms of high blood sugar that suggest GDM, a glucose challenge and/or an oral glucose tolerance test will be performed.

The Glucose Challenge

The glucose challenge is aptly named, because it is indeed a challenge to drink the 50 grams of sugary-sweet glucose that you must consume as part of the test. One hour after you've drunk the Glucola solution, your blood is drawn. If your serum glucose levels are over 135 to 140 mg/dl or higher (7.8 mmol/l), it's an indication that your insulin may not be doing the job it's supposed to, and a three-hour glucose tolerance test is ordered.

The Oral Glucose Tolerance Test (OGTT)

If it was a challenge to drink 50 grams of Glucola, it is a true test of your tolerance (not to mention your intestinal fortitude) to drink the 100 grams of the stuff required for the OGTT. This test is usually administered in the morning because it requires an eight- to fourteen-hour fast before it is performed. Your blood is taken before you are given the Glucola to drink, and then blood is drawn at one hour, two hours, and three hours later.

Fasting levels of 95 mg/dl (5.3 mmol/l) or higher before the test, 180 mg/dl (10 mmol/l) or higher at one hour, 155 mg/dl (8.6 mmol/l) or higher at two hours, and 140 mg/dl (7.8 mmol/l) at three hours suggest GDM. If two or more of these readings are elevated, GDM is diagnosed.

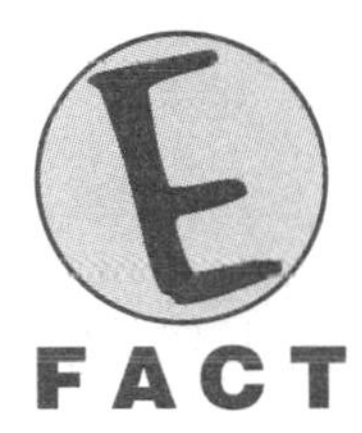

FACT

According to the ADA, women who are obese (a BMI of over 30) and have GDM may benefit from restricting their carbohydrate intake to 35 to 40 percent of their total calories. Studies have shown this can improve fetal outcomes and reduce hyperglycemia.

Back to School

If you're diagnosed with GDM, your first order of business will be meeting with a certified diabetes educator (CDE) and a registered dietitian (RD) to develop an eating and treatment plan. In addition to teaching you about blood glucose testing and other basics of managing your gestational diabetes, they can help you with strategies for dealing with morning sickness and other unique challenges of pregnancy.

Your health care provider can refer you to both a CDE and an RD, and the costs of consultation with both are covered by most health care insurers (although you should check with your specific carrier to find out more about your coverage). If your ob-gyn doesn't offer these essential services, be sure to ask. You can find information about choosing a health care team that's right for you in Chapter 5.

Treating GDM

To lower your blood glucose levels and minimize chances of complications for both you and your baby, you may need to make some lifestyle changes, including carefully watching what you eat and staying active.

Learning dietary control of GDM is a challenge because you have a short window of time to learn what you need to know, and you need results fast. But pregnant women are what doctors like to call "highly motivated patients." That means that like most mothers, you'll do just about anything to ensure your baby has the best possible start in life. So you start blood testing in earnest, learning the lingo of carbohydrate counting, and read volumes on diabetes care.

Again, a good CDE and RD are worth their weight in gold when it comes to learning about food and gestational diabetes. They will explain the basics of carbohydrate counting and coach you on the intricacies of portion estimates, smart restaurant choices, your specific caloric and nutrient needs as a pregnant woman, and more. It also helps to have a good reference book or two around to refer to when you don't have your educator in front of you. Chapters 10 and 11 explain these issues and medical nutrition therapy (MNT) for diabetes in detail.

It's reassuring to know that many women with GDM are able to control their glucose levels through diet and exercise alone, but it's often that second word—exercise—that throws women into a panic. You should know that anything that gets your heart pumping and your body moving is good, and can lower blood glucose levels. That could be as simple as working in your garden or playing with your daughter at the park. If you need motivation, many health clubs, community centers, and hospitals offer prenatal exercise classes. Your health care provider can give you a referral.

And for those who like a more solitary form of fitness, walking is a good way to ease into a workout routine. It's cheap, easy, and always accessible. Even if you live in an inhospitable climate for outdoor walking, you can find a local mall or an indoor track to lap. If you've always been active, then you may be given the green light to do something a little more challenging. Always talk to your doctor first before starting any new fitness activity during pregnancy.

Tracking Your Blood Glucose

Checking your blood glucose levels frequently with a portable home monitor is also an important part of your treatment program. This quick and simple test involves pricking your finger with a fine needle, called a lancet, and placing a small blood drop on a test strip that is inserted into a blood glucose monitor, or meter. The monitor analyzes the amount of glucose in the blood sample and displays the reading. (Chapter 7 has more information on how and when to test your blood glucose levels.)

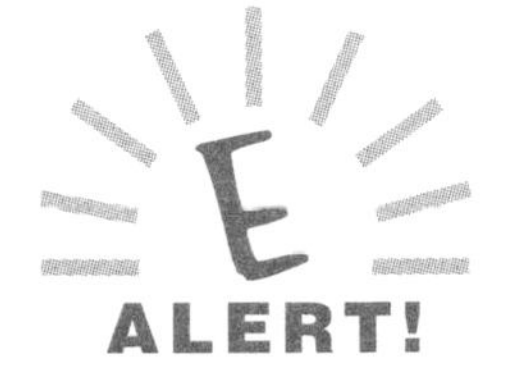

Although the thought of "sticking yourself" repeatedly is a deterrent to many when they first start checking glucose levels, keep in mind that with today's ultrafine lancets, the procedure is relatively painless. If you're experiencing a lot of pain or are having trouble getting a blood sample, take your meter and your technique to your CDE, who can offer you pointers on less painful testing.

When you first get started, you may be testing more frequently as you try to get a handle on how different foods and activities affect your glucose levels. Testing is usually recommended early in the morning before breakfast (fasting test) and after meals (postprandial test). Postprandial tests are taken one hour after the start of your meal, and can be taken again at the two-hour mark. You should keep a written log of all your results (see Chapter 7 for a sample log page). If you exercise regularly, test your glucose levels before and after your workout.

Blood Glucose Target Levels in Women with Gestational Diabetes as Recommended by the ADA

Test	Range
Fasting whole blood glucose	≤95 mg/dl (5.3 mmol/l)
Fasting plasma glucose	≤105 mg/dl (5.8 mmol/l)
1 hour postprandial whole blood glucose	≤140 mg/dl (7.8 mmol/l)
1 hour postprandial plasma glucose	≤155 mg/dl (8.6 mmol/l)
2 hour postprandial whole blood glucose	≤120 mg/dl (6.7 mmol/l)
2 hour postprandial plasma glucose	≤130 mg/dl (7.2 mmol/l)

Ketone Testing

In addition to blood glucose monitoring, your doctor may ask you to perform ketone testing at home. This is done by dipping a ketone test strip in a urine sample. Home monitors that check for blood ketones are also available. Ketones can be a sign that your blood glucose is too high and your body is breaking down fat stores for energy instead of glucose. They can also occur in cases of severe morning sickness if you aren't keeping adequate food down. If you test positive for ketones, call your health care provider right away for further directions.

When You Need Insulin

If you're unable to keep your blood glucose levels down to a safe level with dietary and activity changes only, your doctor may suggest insulin therapy. Oral medications aren't recommended because of the possible risks to the fetus, but insulin does not cross the placenta and is therefore considered safe for you and your developing baby.

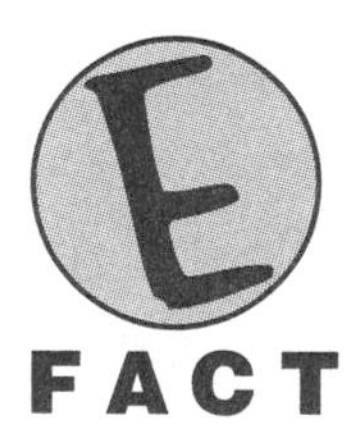

FACT

In 2000, a clinical trial published in the *New England Journal of Medicine* found that the diabetes drug glyburide was as effective as insulin in controlling blood glucose levels in women with GDM. As of early 2003, the drug was not approved for the treatment of GDM by the FDA, however.

Another trip back to the CDE may be in order to teach you how to take insulin and to learn the signs and symptoms of hypoglycemia (low blood sugar). He or she can also work with you to help you understand how to interpret your blood glucose readings and manage your insulin accordingly. Always bring your blood glucose log with you on both your ob-gyn and CDE appointments so you don't have to rely on your memory and so your providers have a more accurate clinical picture on which to base treatment decisions.

Needing to take insulin does not mean you've "failed" at managing your GDM. Consider it another method of ensuring your baby the best possible birth outcome.

How GDM Affects the Baby

Just like babies born to mothers with type 1 or type 2 diabetes, newborns from mothers with GDM can experience hypoglycemia at birth. Low levels of calcium and magnesium in your baby's blood may also be a problem. Jaundice, a yellowing of the skin that happens when your baby has excess bilirubin in his system, may also occur in GDM babies.

Fortunately, all of these conditions are usually easily correctable. And the fact that your GDM has been diagnosed means that your health care team can anticipate these possible problems and diagnose and treat them quickly. You may also have a neonatologist, a doctor that treats high-risk infants, in the delivery room to care for your baby.

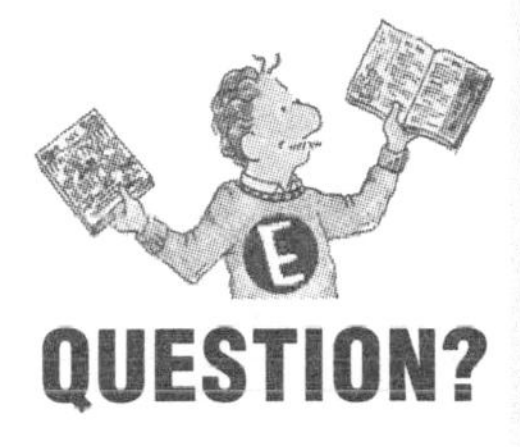

QUESTION?

We had our "birth plan" all finished and were ready to bring it to our doctor, but now that I have GDM, I'm thinking, why bother? Am I right?

Having GDM doesn't mean that all your wishes are automatically thrown out the window. A written agenda of what you want out of your labor and delivery may be even more important when you know interventions may be required. Your doctor can work with you to adjust your plan to reflect appropriate expectations. To learn more about birth plans, check *The Everything® Pregnancy Book, Second Edition* (Adams Media, 2003).

Fetal Macrosomia

Fetal macrosomia, or a baby who is too big for its term, can occur in women with GDM if their blood glucose levels aren't well controlled. Since your blood glucose crosses the placenta and passes into the fetal circulation, your baby will start to produce more and more insulin to counteract its effects. Even the most active baby can't burn off all that glucose (there's only so much room to move around in there). As a result, the extra glucose is stored as fat.

If an ultrasound reveals that your fetus is measuring substantially big for date, macrosomia may be suspected. If your child develops macrosomia, she may become too large to fit through the birth canal, and a C-section may be required. This is another reason why good control of your GDM is so important during pregnancy.

There is also a risk of macrosomia for women who deliver past thirty-eight weeks. For this reason, labor may be induced or a C-section may be scheduled at the thirty-eighth week of gestation. Talk with your doctor early about her thoughts on these interventions to work toward a birth experience that's acceptable for both of you and promotes the best possible outcome for your baby.

Beyond Pregnancy

After you've delivered, you'll have to remain vigilant about your and your child's health. When you visit your doctor for your postpartum evaluation, your glucose levels will once again be tested. If the results indicate impaired glucose tolerance (IGT or prediabetes), you will need to be tested annually for diabetes. If glucose levels are normal, you only require testing once every three years after delivery.

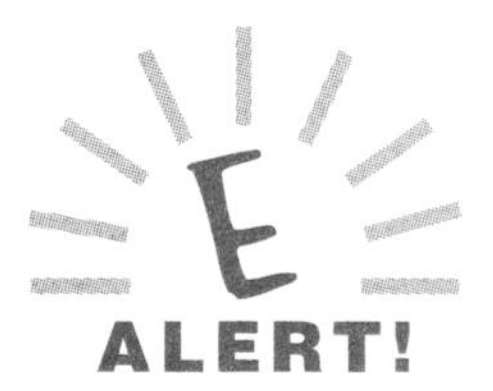

Make sure your primary-care physician gets a copy of all your medical and postpartum records from your ob-gyn and is aware of your history of GDM. If you ever require prescription medications that promote insulin resistance or cause hyperglycemia, it's important that your doctor is aware of your health history.

Long-Term Risks to Mom

One bout with gestational diabetes increases your risk for GDM in subsequent pregnancies, and also increases your long-term risk of developing type 2 diabetes. The good news is that the nutritional skills and exercise habits you pick up during GDM treatment are your best defense against type 2 diabetes, and your doctor will encourage you to continue to use them after delivery. Studies have shown that minor lifestyle changes and weight loss can make a big difference in lowering your insulin resistance.

Another thing you learned in pregnancy—awareness of highs and lows—should not be forgotten after baby's birth. Remember what high blood glucose levels felt like, and if you ever develop the symptoms, see your doctor immediately.

If and when you do decide to become pregnant again, schedule a preconception visit with your ob-gyn to assess your health status, screen for diabetes, and ensure you get your next pregnancy off to a good start.

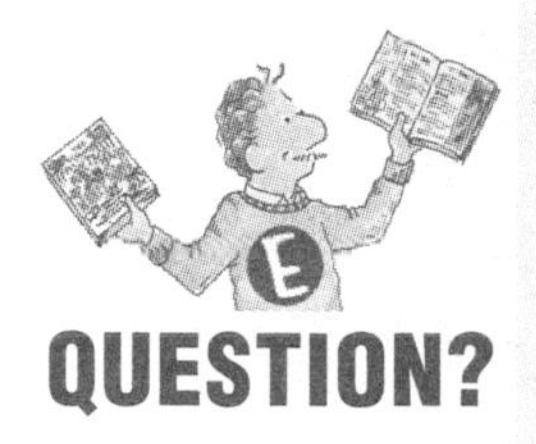

QUESTION?

Is it okay to breastfeed after GDM?
Yes! In addition to all the known benefits breastmilk and nursing offer your baby, breastfeeding may actually kick-start your pancreas, improving beta cell function and lowering your risk of developing type 2 diabetes. Breastfeeding also burns extra calories (about 800 daily) and can help you lose excess pregnancy weight.

Long-Term Risks to Baby

Your new healthy lifestyle should also be something that carries over to your family life. Your child will be at an increased risk for obesity and diabetes as she grows into adolescence and adulthood. The best way to help her is to encourage and model good habits now that will last a lifetime.

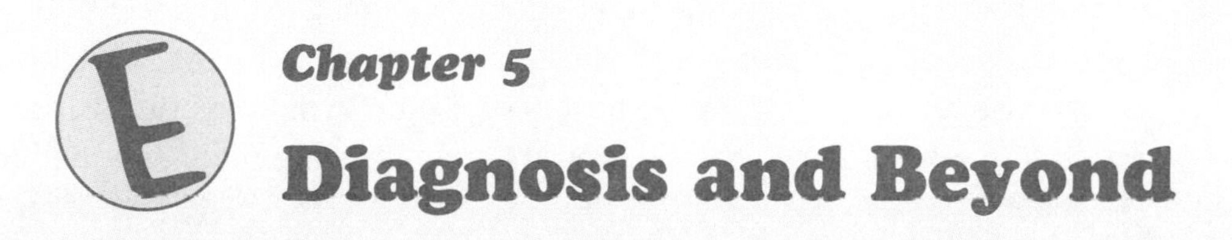

Chapter 5
Diagnosis and Beyond

A diagnosis of diabetes is a scary thing, but having a health care team that is knowledgeable and communicative can make the ride a little less bumpy. Your doctor is only one part of the equation in diabetes—because diabetes is a systemic disease you'll also be seeing a team of specialists to help prevent and treat complications. Choose them thoughtfully and play an active and educated role in your care and you'll be in charge of your diabetes rather than the other way around.

Making the Diagnosis

Diabetes is diagnosed through a lab test that measures the level of glucose in your blood. Because a rise in blood sugar levels might be attributable to some other factor, such as illness or stress, a second blood test is usually performed the following day to establish the diagnosis.

There are actually three different types of diagnostic blood tests in use: the fasting plasma glucose test, casual plasma glucose, and the oral glucose tolerance test. In the absence of overt symptoms or a hyperglycemic crisis, two tests taken on different days are recommended to confirm the diagnosis.

Fasting Plasma Glucose Test (FPG)

The FPG is a carbohydrate metabolism test that measures plasma (blood) glucose levels after a fast of at least eight hours. Fasting stimulates the release of the hormone glucagon, which in turn raises plasma glucose levels by triggering the breakdown of glycogen (stored glucose) in the liver. In people without diabetes, the body will produce and process insulin to counteract this rise in glucose levels. With diabetes, this does not happen, and the tested glucose levels will remain high.

The fasting plasma glucose test should be administered in the morning. Blood glucose tests given in the afternoon tend to provide lower readings and could miss some cases of IGT and diabetes.

According to ADA clinical practice guidelines, a fasting reading of 126 mg/dl (7.0 mmol/l) or higher indicates diabetes, and a second test on a different day should be performed to confirm the diagnosis. If test results are less than 126 mg/dl (7.0 mmol/l) but symptoms of diabetes are present, a follow-up oral glucose tolerance test should be performed.

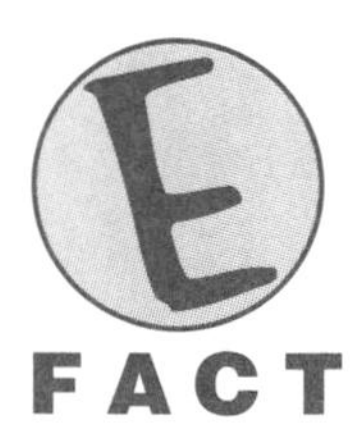

FACT

The normal range for the FPG is considered under 110 mg/dl (6.1 mmol/l). Individuals with FPG results between 110 mg/dl and 125 mg/dl, or a two-hour glucose level rising to 140 to 199 mg/dl (7.8 to 11.0 mmol/l), are said to have impaired glucose tolerance (IGT) or impaired fasting glucose (IFG), also known as prediabetes.

Oral Glucose Tolerance Test (OGTT)

The OGTT is a test that measures blood glucose at hour intervals over a three-hour period. The patient is given a 75-gram drink of glucose solution (Glucola), which should cause glucose levels to rise in the first hour, and then fall back to normal within three hours as the body produces more insulin to normalize glucose levels.

Blood drawn two hours after drinking the glucose solution (also called two-hour postload blood draw) that has glucose levels of under 140 mg/dl (7.8 mmol/l) is considered normal. Two-hour postload levels of 140 mg/dl (7.8 mmol/l) or higher but less than 200 mg/dl (11.1 mmol/l) are an indication of impaired glucose tolerance. Blood glucose levels of 200 mg/dl (11.1 mmol/l) or higher two-hour postload point to diabetes, and should be confirmed by a second OGTT or FPG test on a different day.

Random or Casual Plasma Glucose Test

The random plasma glucose test, also called a casual plasma glucose test, can be given at any time of the day, regardless of whether the patient has eaten or not. Casual plasma glucose levels of 200 mg/dl (11.1 mmol/l) or higher, along with symptoms of diabetes is considered diagnostic of diabetes. A second FPG or OGTT test on another day is recommended to confirm the diagnosis.

ADA Guidelines for Diagnosing Diabetes

Test	Normal Levels	Impaired Glucose Tolerance	Diabetes*
Fasting Plasma Glucose	<110 mg/dl (6.1 mmol/l)	≥110 (6.1 mmol/l) and <126 mg/dl (7.0 mmol/l)	≥126 mg/dl (7.0 mmol/l)
Oral Glucose Tolerance Test**	<140 mg/dl (7.8 mmol/l)	≥140 (7.8 mmol/l) and <200 mg/dl (11.1 mmol/l)	≥200 mg/dl (11.1 mmol/l)
Casual Plasma Glucose			≥200 mg/dl (11.1 mmol/l) in the presence of symptoms

*Diagnosis should be confirmed with an FPG or OGTT on a different day
**Two-hour postload readings

After a diagnosis is made, further lab tests may be ordered to determine the progression of your disease and the possibility of coexisting conditions that are common in diabetes.

C-Peptide Test

If you have, or your doctor suspects you have, type 1 diabetes, a c-peptide test may be ordered. C-peptide is a by-product of insulin. The levels of c-peptide in your bloodstream can help establish how much insulin your pancreas is still able to produce.

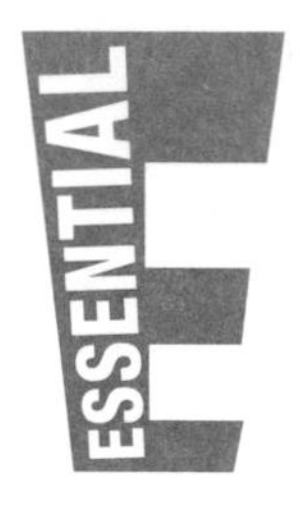

If you are considering going on an insulin pump, a c-peptide test may be ordered. As of 2003, Medicare regulations required a fasting c-peptide level of "less than or equal to 110 percent of the lower limit of normal of the laboratory's measurement method" for coverage of insulin pumps and related supplies.

C-peptide can also diagnose hyperinsulinemia (overproduction of insulin by the pancreas) in type 2 diabetes. If you have had type 2 diabetes for some time, your physician may prescribe the test to determine if your beta cells are still functioning. The normal range for c-peptide levels varies, as there are several different laboratory methods of performing the test; ask your physician for assistance in interpreting your specific results.

Conditions such as pregnancy or renal failure can affect c-peptide levels, as can certain medications and alcohol intake. Also, the test should not be performed immediately following a glucose tolerance test (GTT), as a GTT can artificially elevate c-peptide levels.

Other Tests

If you are a new patient, your physician should take a detailed medical history at your initial visit. A thorough, head-to-toes physical examination to check for the presence of possible complications of diabetes will also be undertaken. This will include an evaluation of your cardiac (heart) function, blood pressure, and a neurological examination of your reflexes, muscle strength, and sensitivity to stimulation.

A monofilament test, which involves touching the bottom of your foot with a piece of fiber resembling a thick strand of fishing line, is a easy and inexpensive way to establish if you have lost sensation in your feet due to nerve damage—a condition called peripheral neuropathy.

Your feet will also be examined carefully for infection, ulceration, and circulatory problems. A weak pedal pulse (pulse taken on the foot) is an early sign of peripheral vascular disease, or PVD, a condition where some blood vessels outside of the heart become narrowed or blocked and, as a result, blood flow is reduced to the surrounding tissues—often the hands and feet. For more information on monofilament testing, PVD, neuropathy, and other complications of diabetes, see Chapter 15.

Other tests that may be performed at or shortly following your initial diagnosis include:

- A urine test for microalbumin, a protein that can indicate problems with kidney function
- An HbA1c blood test, to see what your three-month blood glucose average is
- A fasting blood lipid profile, to check cholesterol levels
- A TSH (thyroid-stimulating hormone) test, to check for thyroid dysfunction, a common risk for people with type 1 diabetes
- Electrocardiogram (ECG), to assess cardiac function

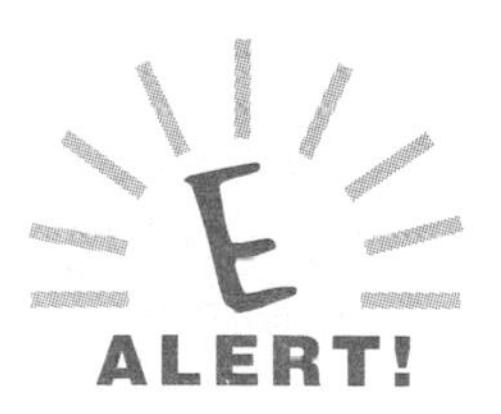

Additional tests and procedures may also be indicated, depending on your specific medical history. Chapter 6 has extensive information on laboratory tests for diabetes and diabetes-related complications.

Choosing a Doctor

Once you have a confirmed diagnosis, it's time to take a step back and make a decision about who will be your partner in managing your diabetes. If you have a doctor who communicates well, listens to your thoughts and concerns, and seems up to speed on current developments in diabetes care, you may decide to stay with her. However, if your doctor-patient relationship is more on the dysfunctional side, it may be time to shop around for someone new. Here are a few questions to consider:

- Does your physician provide cutting edge care? Is he current on the latest clinical studies, new products, and treatment guidelines?
- Is your doctor willing to listen and learn? Does he let you voice questions and concerns without interruption and give you a chance to ask follow-up questions?
- Is she reasonably available? How does she handle daytime and after-hours phone calls from patients? Does she return calls in a timely manner?
- Does he treat the person, not just the disease? Does his treatment philosophy reflect a good understanding of the social and emotional impact of diabetes?
- What's her bedside manner like? Is she abrupt with her staff? Does she brush off patient questions? Do you want a person who just isn't nice to be your treatment partner for the lifelong commitment of diabetes management?
- Does he tell it like it is? Having a doctor who explains tests and treatment decisions is essential. He should be able to communicate with you frankly and in terms you can understand.

Remember, your doctor is only one member of your health care team, albeit an important one. She should communicate well with other members of the team as well as with you—sharing information and getting consultation on treatment decisions when appropriate (for instance, talking with a neonatologist or ob-gyn to discuss a patient that has type 1 diabetes and is pregnant).

Do You Need a Specialist?

You may need to get a new doctor who specializes in diabetes if your health care picture is complex or you or your physician don't feel comfortable with his level of expertise in diabetes care. An endocrinologist is a physician who specializes in gland and hormone disorders. He may work with a variety of endocrine disorders or focus specifically on diabetes. *Diabetologist* is another name for a physician—endocrinologist or otherwise—who specializes in diabetes care. Children with diabetes may also benefit from the expertise of a pediatric endocrinologist if their pediatrician has little to no experience with diabetes.

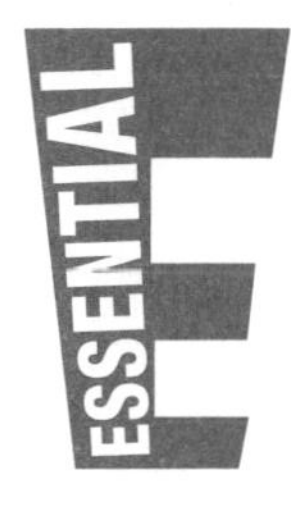

Many people with diabetes continue to see a general practitioner after diagnosis. As long as your doctor has experience treating diabetes, stays up-to-date on the latest in diabetes care, is a partner rather than a dictator in your treatment, and communicates well, it really doesn't matter what abbreviation follows her name.

Communication Is Key

So exactly what defines good communication? It's talking with one another rather than at one another—listening instead of just hearing, and explaining rather than commanding. If you ask your doctor why he has ordered a certain test, he should be able to explain it in laymen's terms. And if your doctor has questions about your self-care, you should be forthright and honest so he can provide you with the best care possible. Here are a few other suggestions you may find useful in improving communication with your doctor:

- Think about the symptom(s), questions, and treatment issues you want to discuss in advance. Bring notes if necessary.
- Bring your medications (in their original bottles) with you. This should include herbs and supplements—your doctor should know what you're taking because some supplements may interact with other medications or may be inappropriate for diabetes patients.
- Treat your doctor as you would like to be treated—respectfully and candidly.
- Bring someone else along to join you after the examination to hear what the doctor is recommending.
- Take your pills as prescribed, and if you are not, let your doctor know so you can discuss an alternative.
- Don't be a "no-show" for appointments, and let the scheduler know exactly what you need to see the doctor for so she can book your appointment for an adequate length of time.

Your Health Care Team

Diabetes is a systemic disease that has the potential to impact every part of your body, so preventative care by a team of trained experts and specialists is an absolute essential.

Your primary-care physician may be able to provide initial screening for diabetes-related complications, but she may also refer you to another doctor who has specialized training in the area of concern. Endocrinologists, diabetologists, internists, ophthalmologists, mental health providers, nephrologists, and podiatrists are just a few of the other care providers that can help you stay healthy and avoid complications.

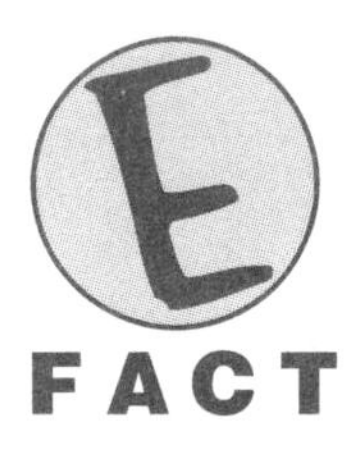

FACT

The Health Insurance Portability Accountability Act (HIPAA) of 1996 provides U.S. patients with access to their medical records upon request within 30 days. Additional state laws governing patient access to medical records and tests results may also apply. Some providers may charge a fee to cover the costs of copying and retrieving patient files. Check with the department of health in your state for the regulations in your area.

Ophthalmologists

The blood vessel damage associated with diabetes puts you at risk for diabetic retinopathy and other vision problems. Ideally, you should see an MD trained in eye diseases—an ophthalmologist—to treat existing eye disease and to screen for problems. An optometrist (an eye care professional who is not a physician) may also screen for diabetic retinopathy. The ADA recommends an annual dilated-eye exam for all people with type 1 and type 2 diabetes (after age ten).

Mental Health Professionals

The psychological toll of diabetes can also be a tremendous burden, both emotionally and physically. Up to 20 percent of people living with diabetes also suffer from depression. Therapists, psychiatrists, psychologists, and/or trained counselors can help you cope with the stresses of diabetes;

support groups are also a great resource for coming to grips with diabetes and learning from the experiences of others.

Nephrologists

Because diabetes is the number one cause of chronic kidney disease, you may see a nephrologist—a physician specializing in renal care. If kidney disease progresses to ESRD (end-stage renal disease), a nephrologist will also be in charge of prescribing dialysis treatments.

Podiatrists

Proper foot care and regular exams of the feet are extremely important in diabetes care, so a podiatrist, or foot doctor, is also a key member of the health care team. Podiatrists can detect and treat neuropathy (nerve damage) of the feet and foot ulcers. They can also help educate patients on preventative foot care.

Other Team Players

Other specialists that may be on your health care team include the following:

- **Gastroenterologist:** A physician who specializes in diseases and disorders of the digestive tract.
- **Gynecologist:** A doctor specializing in women's reproductive medicine.
- **Obstetrician:** A physician who monitors pregnancy and birth.
- **Urologist:** An MD with special training in treating the urinary tract.
- **Neurologist:** A specialist of the central nervous system (CNS), who treats CNS disorders as well as those of the peripheral nervous system, such as neuropathy.
- **Dermatologist:** A doctor who treats skin diseases and disorders, and may have special training in wound care.
- **Physical therapist:** A trained health care professional who assists in strength and mobility recovery through exercise and other techniques.

Coordinating Care

With an army of specialists treating your diabetes and related complications, communication is essential. In an ideal world, all of your doctors would follow up with your primary physician quickly and consult with another specialist promptly when your medical problems extend outside of their area of expertise. In reality, you may face missing lab reports, contradictory treatment recommendations, and other obstacles.

Short of hiring a personal secretary to keep track of your complex medical schedule and rapidly expanding charts, there are a few things you can do to ensure that all your providers are on the same page of the playbook. If your primary provider refers you to a specialist, call forty-eight hours before your appointment to make sure the new physician has all the clinical information she needs from your regular doctor. And when you go to your appointment, ask the specialist what her office procedure is for following up with your primary provider. Here's what else you can do:

- Offer to deliver treatment reports from specialists to your primary-care provider and vice-versa.
- Ask for hard copies of lab results and diagnostic tests so you have a backup and don't waste a trip to the doctor's office if they don't get delivered.
- Keep a running list of all medications that are prescribed by your various physicians and bring it to your doctor appointments.
- Take notes of questions, concerns, and new issues raised at your appointments so you can share them with your primary provider.

Remember, your health care providers work for you, but you are the one ultimately in charge of your own health care. Don't be shy about following up on your treatment, and don't let any doctor or medical staff make you feel guilty about doing so. If they do, it may be time to consider finding someone new.

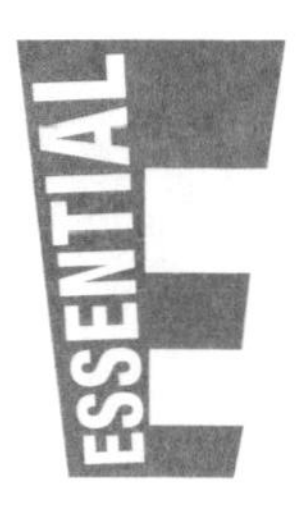

Diabetes education classes are usually geared toward the newly diagnosed, although there are some "refresher" courses for people who have lived with diabetes for some time or who want to learn ways of tightening their blood glucose control.

Getting a Good Education

Since you spend most of your time away from the doctor's office, it's important to learn as much as you can about how you can manage your diabetes and prevent complications at home. In fact, diabetes is such a complex disease that it merits its own course of study. Self-care, a generalized term for looking after yourself and promoting wellness, is the main thrust of diabetes education. You'll also learn essential skills like testing blood glucose levels and injecting insulin.

Going to School

Your doctor can refer you to classes in your area and, in fact, should offer you information on diabetes education at or shortly following diagnosis. Classes are often held at local hospitals or freestanding clinics, and are typically covered by most health insurance plans (check with your insurer on your eligibility).

Diabetes classes cover a wide range of issues, including how diabetes affects your body physically and emotionally, how to test blood sugars, the importance of exercise, knowing the signs of a blood sugar emergency, regulating medications and/or insulin, recognizing and preventing complications, and coping with lifestyle issues. Another primary teaching point is how to manage your diet with diabetes.

There are also CDEs who work one-on-one with patients. Again, your doctor can provide a referral, or you can contact the American Association of Diabetes Educators to locate a CDE in your area (see Appendix A for more information).

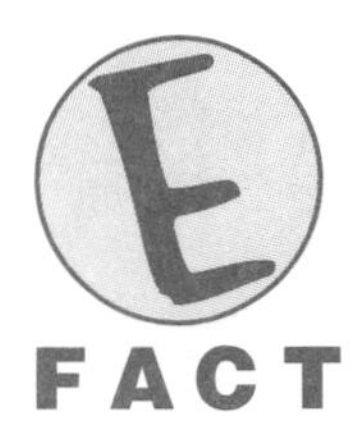
FACT

Diabetes education classes are typically taught by a diabetes nurse educator who is usually a certified diabetes educator (CDE). Educators with the CDE designation have completed specific training in diabetes patient education. Classes range from short workshops to intensive, multipart courses.

Food Savvy RDs

Dietary management is one of the cornerstones of diabetes care, especially in type 2 diabetes where weight loss may also be an issue. A registered dietitian (RD) or a nutritionist who works with patients with diabetes is an essential part of your care team.

An RD can teach you concepts like carbohydrate counting and dietary exchanges, and explain how certain foods affect blood glucose levels. Most important, your dietitian can also work with you one-on-one to design a meal plan that fits your particular lifestyle. If you're a vegetarian, it will do you little good to get a cookie-cutter fish and meat menu. And if you have a job that keeps you out on the road a great deal of the time, you need someone who can help you make healthy choices outside of the kitchen. Consulting with an RD allows you to develop menus based in reality. If your diet is practical, you're more likely to follow it and stick to it in the long term.

Taking Control

In diabetes-care lingo, control is maintaining blood glucose levels as close to normal (nondiabetic) levels as much of the time as possible. The American Diabetes Association recommends that people with diabetes aim for blood sugar levels of 80 to 120 mg/dl before meals and 100 to 140 mg/dl at bedtime.

It is important to remember that the ADA target goals are general recommendations only, and you will work with your doctor to determine the blood glucose goals that are right for you and your particular health picture. If you haven't figured it out already, while there are many guidelines and targets in diabetes care, in practice just about everything about the disease varies by individual. A food that sends one person's blood sugar off the charts may cause barely a ripple for another.

Is your head spinning yet? With all the information thrown at you, both in class and by well-meaning friends and relatives (who quite frequently spread misinformation rather than fact), being overwhelmed is completely normal. Take a deep breath and remember three things:

1. You aren't in this alone–your health care team is there to help.
2. You don't have to learn it all at once–control involves some trial and error.
3. Reinventing the wheel is not necessary–others have gone before you, and you'll find getting through the physical and emotional demands much easier if you join a support group and draw on their wisdom.

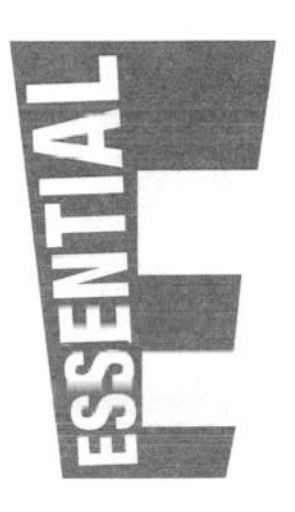

Frequent blood glucose testing, careful monitoring of what and how much you eat, exercise, and other lifestyle adjustments are the paths to achieve control. In some cases, "power tools" like oral medications or insulin may also be necessary.

A Treatment Triad

Treatment for the disease won't be as simple as filling your prescription and getting back to business as usual. People living with type 1 diabetes will rely on insulin as their main weapon against complications, but diet and exercise also play an important role.

Those with type 2 diabetes may be able to use diet and exercise to effectively keep their blood sugar levels under control. Often, a little help from oral medications or insulin is also required. If you need medication to control your diabetes, that doesn't make you any less successful at managing your disease than someone who has been able to do it through diet and exercise only. Together, diet, exercise, and medication are simply different tools designed to help you achieve the same goal—normalized blood glucose levels.

Eat Right

If you have type 1 diabetes, what you eat determines how much insulin your body requires, so knowing how food choices impact your blood sugar is essential.

Because over 80 percent of people with type 2 diabetes are overweight or obese, eating for both blood sugar control and weight loss is often a fundamental component of type 2 care. Appropriate food choices and dietary considerations for diabetes, also called medical nutrition therapy (or MNT), are covered in detail in Chapter 11.

Exercise

Exercise is fundamental to good health and well-being. It lowers blood glucose levels, improves heart health, and promotes weight loss in overweight people with type 2 diabetes. However, people with diabetes do need to take precautions with their exercise routine to ensure that they don't experience a hypoglycemic episode. Chapter 12 has further details on getting fit with diabetes.

Medication

While some people are able to successfully manage their type 2 diabetes through diet and exercise, many others require the additional assistance of oral medications. Turn to Chapter 9 for detailed descriptions of prescription drugs used in type 2 treatment.

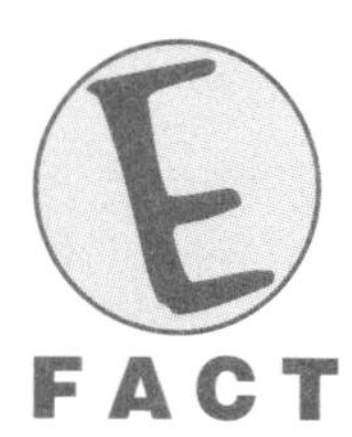

FACT

Both the American Diabetes Association (ADA) and the American Association of Clinical Endocrinologists (AACE) have issued clinical practice recommendations that U.S. providers look to as professional guidelines for diagnosis and treatment. See Appendix C for an overview of preventative care standards.

Chapter 6

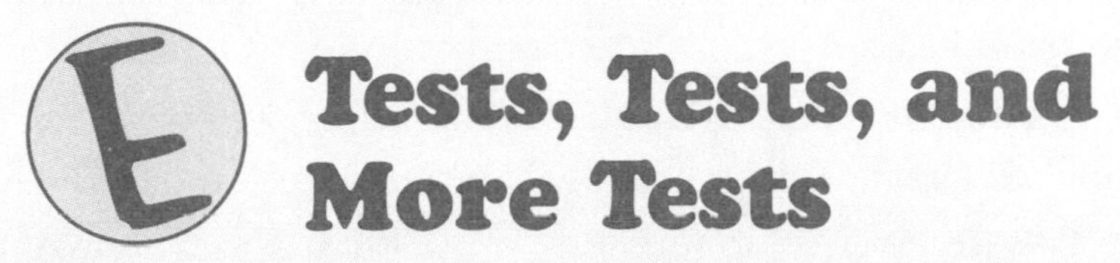

Tests, Tests, and More Tests

The average person with diabetes racks up $13,243 in medical care annually, compared to $2,560 for people without diabetes. Although the price tag sounds high, the toll of uncontrolled blood glucose levels and associated complications is much higher. Think of all the prescriptions, lab work, and doctor's visits as preventative maintenance. Like spending money to restore a vintage car, your investment will pay big dividends in smooth operation and enjoyment later.

The HbA1c Test

In addition to your self-monitoring routine (covered in the next chapter), you'll be donating quite a bit of blood to the testing cause at your doctor's office. One of the most important of these tests is the glycosylated hemoglobin test (also called a glycated hemoglobin test, GHB, HbA1c, or simply A1c). The A1c assesses your long-term, three-month glucose average.

Glycosylated hemoglobin is a substance produced when excess glucose attaches itself to hemoglobin (a substance in red blood cells). The higher your percentage of glycated hemoglobin, the higher your blood glucose levels were over the past ninety-day period.

The ADA recommends that an A1c be performed at least twice annually, and up to four times a year for individuals who are undergoing adjustments to treatment or failing to meet treatment goals. Patients who use insulin to control their type 1 or type 2 diabetes should have the test performed quarterly as well.

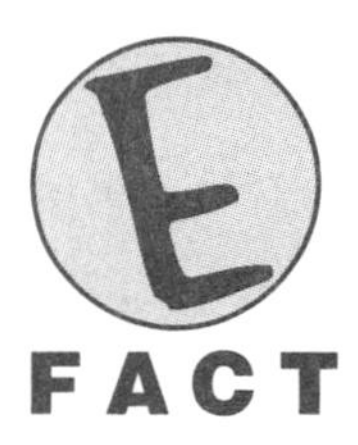

FACT

There are different laboratory methods of measuring glycosylated hemoglobin, depending on the subtype of hemoglobin measured. If your HbA1c levels suddenly change for no apparent reason, ask your doctor if he or she has changed labs or lab methods that could affect the interpretation of your test results.

Long-Term Control

A1c levels are the best measure of how you're doing in the long term. While home monitoring offers you a single snapshot of where your blood sugar is at a particular point in time, an A1c test is like a surveillance camera running for three months, day and night, giving you the big picture of your average blood glucose levels.

The Diabetes Control and Complications Trial (DCCT), a landmark clinical study that took place in medical centers across the United States in the early 1990s, demonstrated that people with type 1 diabetes were 40 to 75 percent less likely to develop neuropathy, retinopathy, and nephropathy (kidney disease) when they kept their A1c values as 7.2 percent (achieved through an "intensive care" routine of testing four times daily, keeping in close contact with care providers, and participating in diabetes education courses). Follow-up studies of DCCT participants also found that tight control of blood glucose reduced the risk of atherosclerosis (as measured by carotid artery wall thickness), a benefit that remained six years after the DCCT concluded.

Similarly, the United Kingdom Prospective Diabetes Study (UKPDS), another large-scale study, found that participants with type 2 diabetes who kept their A1c values below 7.0 percent had a 25 percent reduction in the incidence of these same complications. And for every percentage point decrease in HbA1c achieved, there was a 35 percent reduction in the risk of complications. Whether you have type 1 or type 2 diabetes, the A1c is not only a look back at the past three months, but a glimpse into your future risk of complications.

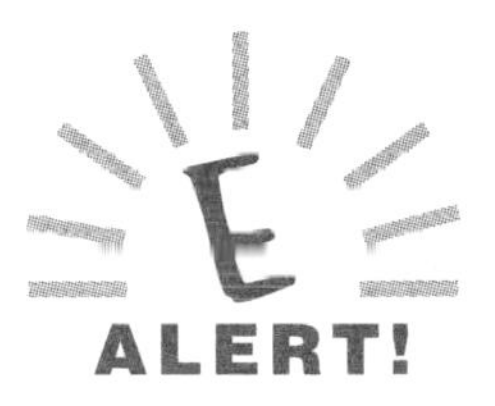

Certain conditions and substances can affect the results of an A1c test. Vitamin C and E, opiates, and salicylates like aspirin can influence results of some A1c tests, as can iron deficiency anemia and chronic alcoholism.

Determining Your Target Goal

People *without* diabetes have an A1c of around 5 percent. It is possible for people with well-controlled diabetes to achieve A1c levels in a range very close to normal. The ADA suggests a <7 percent A1c goal, while the American Association of Clinical Endocrinologists recommends that individuals with diabetes try to achieve a target A1c of ≤6.5 percent to minimize the risk of long-term complications.

Do not be discouraged if your initial A1c tests are higher. Target A1c levels are as individual as diabetes itself. Your doctor will look at your medical history, age, lifestyle, and other factors, and will work with you to define a custom target goal specific to your needs. It can take some time to get your A1c where you want it. The average A1c at time of diagnosis is 10.9 to 15.5 percent, which leaves a lot of room for improvement.

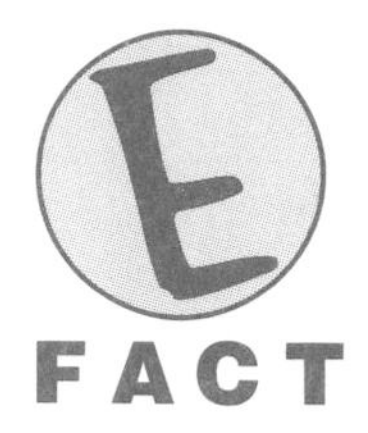

FACT

The FDA approved the A1cNow (Metrika), the first home A1c monitoring blood test, in 2002. The single-use test kit, which is available without a prescription, uses blood from a finger stick, and displays results in eight minutes.

Other Glucose Tests

Your provider may do a random blood glucose test to check the accuracy of your self-monitoring and/or your home meter. She may also test your glucose levels if she is making an adjustment to your medication or treatment routine. Results are provided in plasma glucose values.

The Fructosamine Test

This is another test that measures your blood sugar over a period of time (2 to 3 weeks, as opposed to the 8 to 12 weeks measured by the HbA1c test). The fructosamine test is a measurement of glycated serum proteins, and may be used as a companion to HbA1c when you want to find out how blood glucose control has responded to treatment changes in a shorter time period.

Fructosamine tests are available as home testing kits, but they should not be thought of as a replacement for daily glucose monitoring or HbA1c tests.

Urine Glucose Tests

Available as reagent "dipstick" tests, urinary glucose tests were once the standard method of measuring glucose levels at home for people with diabetes. With the advent of accurate home monitoring systems, urine glucose tests are now usually relegated to the purpose of infrequent screening.

These tests have several drawbacks. First, they are time-delayed—they can't tell you what your blood glucose level is right now, but only several hours later after glucose has filtered into the urine and urine has collected in the bladder and is ready to leave the body. They are also not highly sensitive or specific; a negative urine test can ensure only that your blood glucose levels are below 180 mg/dl, well above a "controlled" range for most people.

Since they are relatively inexpensive, urine glucose tests might be preferred over SMBG (self-monitoring of blood glucose levels) in patients who cannot afford blood-monitoring supplies. They may also be used by patients who can't or won't blood test due to discomfort or other reasons. If you have hypoglycemic unawareness, or are prone to excessive blood sugar lows, it is critical that blood monitoring be used instead of urine monitoring, as urine glucose testing cannot detect blood glucose lows.

What about Insulin Tests?

There are several ways of testing glucose levels, but what about insulin testing? There is a way to test insulin—the insulin serum test, which measures the amount of insulin in the bloodstream. However, given its expense and lack of clinical usefulness, it is rarely used in diabetes diagnosis and assessment.

Insulin has a short half-life and is significantly cleared from the body before it even reaches the general circulation. In addition, the test does not differentiate between injected and endogenous (or self-produced) insulin. Instead of testing insulin, assessing levels of c-peptide, a by-product of insulin and a more accurate predictor of beta cell function, is more common. Chapter 5 has more information on the c-peptide test.

Lipid Profile

Because cardiovascular disease is the leading cause of death among people with diabetes, the ADA recommends an annual fasting lipid panel as part of regular preventative diabetes care. If you are working with your physician to control lipid levels through medication or diet, testing may be done more often.

A fasting lipid profile is a blood test that assesses your risk for developing cardiovascular complications by measuring levels of total cholesterol, high-density lipoprotein (HDL or "good") cholesterol, triglycerides, and low-density lipoprotein (LDL or "bad") cholesterol.

It is also used to diagnose dyslipidemia, a condition characterized by high triglyceride and low HDL cholesterol levels that is common in type 2 diabetes and increases the overall risk of heart disease.

Cholesterol Goals Recommended for Adults with Diabetes

	NCEP* III Guidelines	ADA** Guidelines
HDL	≥40–60 mg/dl	>40 mg/dl (men) >50 mg/dl (women)
LDL	<100 mg/dl	<100 mg/dl
Triglycerides	<150 mg/dl	<150 mg/dl

*The National Cholesterol Education Program
**"Standards of Medical Care for Patients with Diabetes Mellitus,"ADA Position Statement, 2003

Medical history, gender, age, ethnicity, and even geographic region of origin can impact cholesterol levels. Triglyceride levels can be raised by kidney and liver disease and alcoholism. High serum cholesterol levels can be triggered by poor dietary habits, pancreatitis, hypothyroidism, lipid disorders, and certain kidney and liver diseases. High LDL levels put one at an increased risk of coronary artery disease.

More Cardiovascular Tests

The ADA suggests that primary-care physicians assess their patients' heart disease risk factors annually and prescribe cardiac testing accordingly.

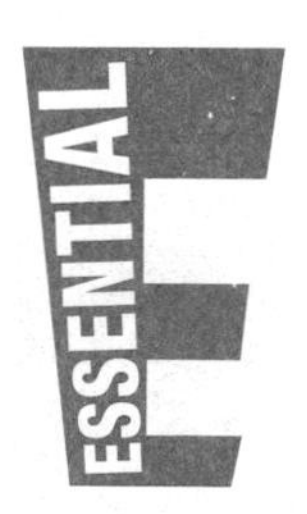

Since an electrocardiogram (ECG) is fairly inexpensive and noninvasive, your physician may perform it on an annual basis or even more frequently, especially if you have a history of heart disease or other additional risk factors besides your diabetes.

Electrocardiogram (ECG, or EKG)

An ECG measures the electrical impulses put out by the heart and creates a visual representation, or tracing, of them. The test is used to check for irregularities in heart rhythm or rate and to detect signs of coronary artery disease.

For a resting ECG, you will be asked to lie flat on a table while sensor patches (leads) are attached to ten various points on the body. The sensors are attached to wires that transfer your heart's electrical impulses into the ECG unit, where a tracing is generated. The test is very brief, taking only about five to ten minutes from start to finish. Your physician will then review the tracing for abnormalities that may indicate an artery blockage or other heart problems.

Exercise Stress Test

As the name implies, an exercise stress test evaluates how your heart and cardiovascular system perform under the pressure of exercise. Your heart is again monitored with ECG leads and a blood pressure cuff. A pulse oximeter (a small, painless clamp that uses light to measure the level of oxygen in your bloodstream) is attached to a finger or other site with sufficient blood flow. Baseline levels of your heart function are taken at rest before the stress test begins.

A stress test is usually performed on a treadmill or stationary bicycle. The level of exertion, or stress, is increased periodically until the patient reaches a specific heart rate. Each time the stress increases, vital signs are measured. The test will be stopped if chest pain, high blood pressure, or other danger signs develop. The whole procedure typically takes about fifteen to twenty minutes, and your heart will continue to be monitored after the exercise portion ends until vital signs return to baseline levels.

Echoes and Scans

Your primary-care provider may also recommend other tests that assess cardiac function and structure, including nuclear perfusion and echocardiography. Nuclear perfusion tests, such as a thallium scan, use a trace amount of radioactive material injected into the bloodstream. The radioactive material is absorbed by cardiac muscle and allows better visualization of the heart structures using a special camera. Poor absorption is associated with inadequate blood flow (perfusion) and may indicate that the arteries leading to that portion of the heart are diseased.

Echocardiography, or "echo," uses ultrasound to create an image of the heart. A small wand, called a transducer, is passed over the chest and sound waves emitted by the transducer bounce off the structures of the heart. The resulting picture is displayed on a video screen. Blood flow is also visible.

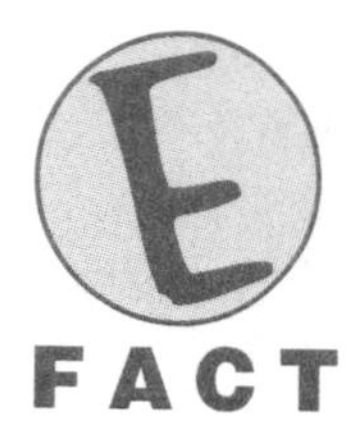

FACT

Both the nuclear perfusion scan and the echo are often performed immediately following a stress test. These noninvasive procedures may be performed by your primary-care provider or by a cardiologist.

Kidney Function Tests

Diabetes is the leading cause of chronic kidney failure, the end stage of renal disease (ESRD). Uncontrolled high glucose levels can damage the nephrons—the filtering units of the kidney that remove excess fluids and waste products from the bloodstream. Regular screening for early signs of kidney problems is an essential part of diabetes care.

Testing for Proteinuria

Healthy kidneys should filter and absorb proteins instead of excreting them into the urine. A proteinuria test detects the presence of protein in the urine—a sign of kidney disease or damage.

A proteinuria test is performed at diagnosis and at least annually thereafter. If you have a history of kidney problems or are at high risk for renal disease, this test may be performed more frequently.

Chemical reagent test strips (dipsticks) may be used to test for protein. They are quick and easy, requiring only a small urine sample and a few minutes for testing. However, a twenty-four-hour urine collection is the gold standard for the proteinuria test. Up to 150 milligrams of protein excreted in a twenty-four-hour period is considered a safe and acceptable level. Moderate levels of protein (0.5 to 4 g/24 hours) are often present in renal disease as a complication of diabetes. High levels (≥3.0-3.5 g/24 hours) occur in nephrotic syndrome. Proteinuria can also signal other urinary tract disorders.

Testing for Microalbuminuria

The microalbumin test checks for another type of protein—albumin—in the urine. The urine test may be random (a spot test at your doctor's office), an overnight collection, or a twenty-four-hour collection. The spot test is typically preferred. It is a more sensitive test than a dipstick protein test, designed to detect microscopic amounts of albumin; the presence of levels of albumin from 30 to 299 milligrams signals high levels of albumin, or microalbuminuria, and is one of the earliest signs of diabetic nephropathy (kidney disease).

Screening for microalbuminuria should be performed annually. If you have type 1 diabetes, current ADA guidelines recommend that testing begin with puberty and/or five years after diagnosis. If you are type 2, screening should start at diagnosis and take place every year thereafter. If microalbumin is present on a test, a repeat test should be performed to confirm the results. For more on diabetic kidney disease, see Chapter 15.

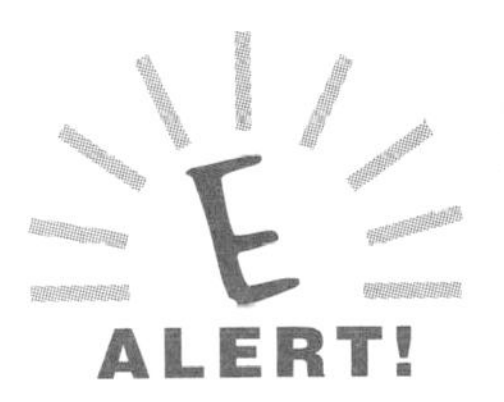

If microalbumin is present on several consecutive tests, it usually indicates diabetic nephropathy, or kidney disease due to diabetes. Bladder infection and/or nephritis can also cause an elevated microalbumin level, as can high blood pressure and periods of hyperglycemia.

Urine Creatinine Clearance

Creatinine clearance measures the kidney's ability to filter creatinine from the blood. Creatinine is a metabolic by-product of creatine, the amino acid that supplies energy for muscle contractions. Normal kidneys should filter creatinine, a waste product, into the urine at a constant rate.

Before a creatinine clearance urine test is performed, a blood sample is taken to determine the level of creatinine in the bloodstream. You are then given a container to collect urine output for twenty-four hours. The final specimen is analyzed for creatinine output, and the creatinine clearance is computed by comparing the urine creatinine to the original blood creatinine levels. If kidney function is impaired, creatinine levels in the urine will be low. The normal range of results for this test are 85 to 146 ml/minute/1.73 m^2 for men and 81 to 134 ml/minute/1.73 m^2 for women.

The ADA may recommend that this test be performed five years after diagnosis in individuals with type 1 diabetes, immediately following diagnosis in people with type 2 diabetes, and at least annually thereafter for both type 1 and type 2. It may be performed more often with those patients at high risk for renal disease.

Low creatinine clearance levels indicate kidney disease (i.e., polycystic kidney disease, glomerulonephritis, renal cancer), congestive heart failure, and/or severe dehydration.

Serum Creatinine

Serum (or blood) creatinine levels may also be measured to assess kidney function. Creatinine is filtered out of the bloodstream by the kidneys. Creatinine blood levels greater than 1.2 mg/dl for women and 1.4 mg/dl for men points to inadequate filtering by the kidneys (renal impairment). Serum creatinine may also be performed as part of a urinary creatinine clearance test.

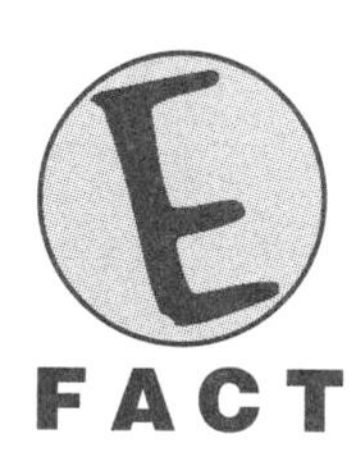

FACT

Can't keep your creatinine straight? Just remember that healthy, functioning kidneys will cleanse this waste product from the blood and move it into the urine for disposal—so serum levels should be low and urine levels should be high.

Blood Urea Nitrogen (BUN)

Urea is another waste product that is filtered from the blood by the kidneys. Urea is generated in the liver by metabolized protein. Your BUN level can help your physician determine your glomerular filtration rate (GFR), or the rate at which your kidneys are filtering waste and fluids from your body. Elevated BUN levels indicate a slowdown in kidney function. Normal adult BUN levels are between 7 and 20 mg/dl. BUN will rise as kidney function falls.

Ketones and Diabetic Ketoacidosis

Ketones are formed when the body can't use insulin to process glucose into fuel and is forced to burn fat for energy. Trace amounts of ketones are not unusual and are usually no cause for alarm, but when accompanied by elevated blood sugars in high enough levels, ketones can trigger diabetic ketoacidosis (DKA), a potentially fatal medical emergency. DKA usually occurs in situations where someone has stopped taking needed insulin injections; is taking an insufficient dose of insulin; or is taking contaminated, expired, or otherwise bad insulin. The physical stress of a flu, cold, or other illness usually increases both blood glucose levels and the need for insulin, and DKA often occurs in these situations.

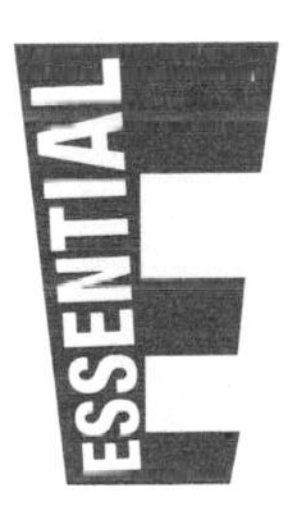

Always check your urine for ketones If your blood glucose levels are 250 mg/dl or higher for two or more consecutive readings. Although people with type 1 diabetes are much more prone to DKA, it is possible for someone with type 2 diabetes to develop it as well. For more on ketone testing and ketoacidosis, see Chapter 14.

If your provider suspects the onset of DKA, she will probably check the level of ketones in your blood. It may also be performed as part of a routine urinalysis. However, there is also a urine test (frequently used at home) to check for the presence of ketones. The test uses a chemically treated reagent strip (Ketostix) that is dipped in a urine sample to check for the presence of ketones. The strip changes color and the color is matched to an enclosed chart that indicates the presence and level of ketones in the urine.

If you have type 1 diabetes, your provider will recommend that you keep a bottle of ketone test strips on hand for home testing. Some people with type 2 diabetes, including children and pregnant women, may also be advised to have ketone test supplies available. In situations where your blood glucose is prone to go high—such as when you are ill—monitoring of urinary ketone levels is essential for preventing ketoacidosis. If testing indicates the presence of moderate or high levels of ketones, you should contact your doctor immediately.

Comprehensive Eye Exam

Diabetes can cause blood vessels in the retina to become damaged or blocked, resulting in vision loss—a condition known as diabetic retinopathy. The National Eye Institute (NEI) estimates that half of all people with diabetes will develop retinopathy at some point in their lifetime. They are also at risk for developing cataracts and glaucoma, which may impair vision.

Both the ADA and the NEI recommend an annual dilated-eye exam for people with diabetes. If you have type 1 diabetes and have no known vision problems, the first exam may be between three and five years following initial diagnosis after age ten; for type 2 diabetes, it should be at or shortly following diagnosis. If you have diagnosed eye disease, you may require more frequent assessment to monitor treatment and disease progression.

In a dilated-eye exam, eyedrops are used to counteract the reflexes that normally trigger the pupil to shrink in bright light. The ophthalmologist uses a high-intensity focused light called a slit-lamp to illuminate the eye. Dilation opens up the pupil, allowing the ophthalmologist to view the back, or fundus, of the retina and the blood vessels and optic nerve situated there.

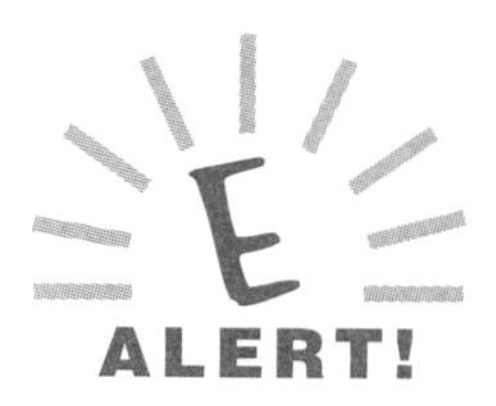

Pregnant women with pre-existing diabetes (not gestational diabetes) should have a dilated-eye examination during the first trimester of pregnancy to screen for microvascular (blood vessel) problems. Additional eye exams may be indicated depending on your medical history and the outcome of the initial exam. The ADA also recommends a preconception eye examination, if possible.

An intraocular pressure test, also called a tonometry test, is used to screen for glaucoma. Tonometry is sometimes called a "puff test" because it may involve blowing a quick puff of air into your eye and measuring the resistance it meets. Another type of pressure test, applanation, uses fluorescein dye to temporarily color the cornea before a tonometer instrument is placed against the eye to measure fluid pressure. Anesthetic drops are used to relieve any discomfort.

Other parts of a comprehensive eye exam may include the following tests:

- **Visual acuity test:** The familiar "big E" Snellen eye chart
- **Visual field test:** A test of your peripheral (side) vision
- **Refraction test:** Checks your ability to see an object at a specific distance
- **Binocular test:** Assesses your eye teamwork—how well the muscle coordination and control of your eyes work in tandem

If you wear glasses or contact lenses, your exam should also include an evaluation of your current prescription. (E)

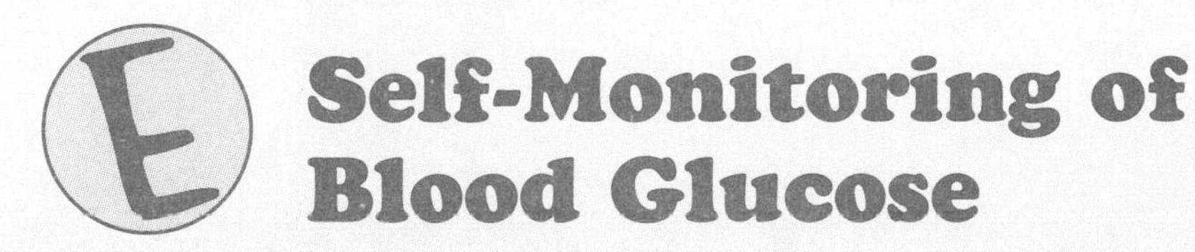

Chapter 7
Self-Monitoring of Blood Glucose

A home blood glucose monitor or meter—a device that analyzes a blood sample and gives you a reading of your current blood sugar levels—is the next best thing to having a lab in your medicine cabinet. Monitors are probably the single most useful tool you have for knowing what's going on with your diabetes, mainly because they are always accessible, provide instant results, and don't require a trip to the doctor's office.

Why Test?

Regular self-monitoring of blood glucose levels (SMBG) gives you a quick clinical snapshot of exactly where your blood glucose levels are at any given moment. Testing, and keeping a detailed log of test results and the circumstances that surround them, will help you understand how certain foods and activities impact your blood sugar. Once you are able to detect patterns in blood glucose changes over time, you can use the information to adjust your treatment accordingly.

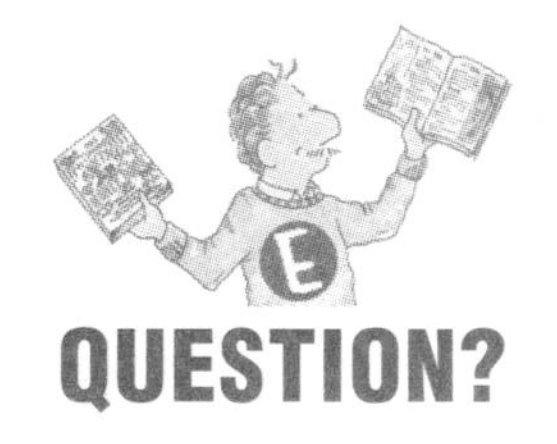

QUESTION?

I can't stand the thought of sticking myself. Can't I just test for sugar in my urine?

You could, but it would do little to help you control your diabetes. Urine glucose testing was the way it was done before home glucose monitors became commonplace. But because urine collects in your bladder for several hours before it leaves the body and only contains glucose when blood levels are over 180 mg/dl, it isn't a very timely or sensitive test. Worse, it cannot help detect potentially dangerous low blood sugar levels.

The Diabetes Control and Complications Trial (DCCT), a landmark clinical study, found that tight control of blood glucose levels using SMBG significantly reduced the risk of diabetes-related complications. Since the study was published in 1993, the ADA has developed guidelines on SMBG and home testing has become a recommended, routine self-care practice.

Another role of SMBG is to help you assess how effective your medication or insulin is in controlling your glucose levels. It is also an invaluable tool for adjusting the timing of medication to ensure the best possible control.

Perhaps most important, SMBG can help you avoid life-threatening blood sugar emergencies. If you are under stress, sick with the flu, or taking medications that affect blood glucose levels, regular testing can help you keep close tabs on your blood sugar levels so you can take action before they go dangerously high.

Testing before, after, and possibly during exercise can help you avoid a precipitous drop in blood glucose levels. It's also wise to test if you've been drinking alcohol, another trigger for hypoglycemia. If you feel a low coming on, a quick test can confirm your levels so you can take action immediately.

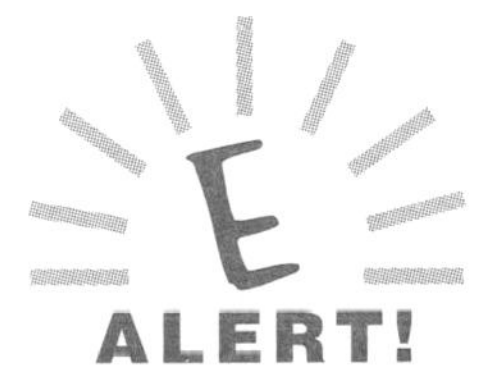

Home glucose testing is particularly important for people with a condition known as *hypoglycemic unawareness*. These individuals have lost the ability to perceive the normal warning signs that blood sugars are dropping too low—such as shakiness, anxiety, sweatiness, hunger, irritability, and rapid heartbeat. Without testing, they may lose consciousness before realizing they are experiencing a hypoglycemic episode.

Developing a Testing Schedule

When to test is a matter of debate. Some people test once when they wake up. Others test up to eight times a day—morning, night, and before and after meals. As a general rule, when your diagnosis is new and you're learning how different factors affect your diabetes, checking your glucose levels frequently is encouraged. The same holds true for monitoring any changes to your treatment routine.

People with type 1 diabetes may need to test more than those with type 2, since they need to use the results to adjust insulin accordingly. And people with glucose levels that fluctuate widely, often without warning (a condition known as *brittle diabetes*), may also need to test more frequently than others.

When determining a schedule for blood glucose testing with your doctor, make sure you discuss any financial or insurance issues that may impact your testing routine. Test strips are expensive (they may cost more than the monitor itself), and some insurance plans put a cap on the quantity of testing supplies they will cover for a given time period. Find out what your insurer offers and work from there. In some cases, your provider may be able to offer you some free product samples to augment your supply.

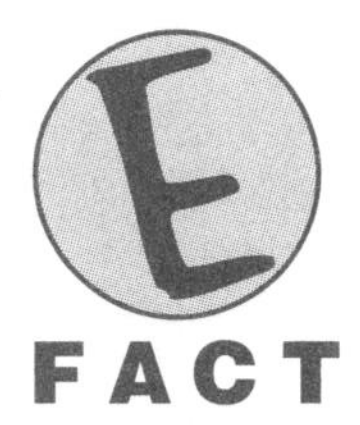

FACT

In the United States, home blood glucose monitors display readings as mg/dl (milligrams over deciliters). However, everywhere else outside the United States, the standard is mmol/l. Some monitors that are sold internationally may have an option for switching back and forth between mg/dl and mmol/l displays.

Target Goals

The ultimate goal is to get blood glucose levels as close to normal as possible. However, if you have hypoglycemic unawareness, or if you have other medical conditions that affect your control, your target glucose levels may be a bit higher. Young children with diabetes who may not yet have the ability to recognize symptoms of hypoglycemia also tend to have slightly higher goals. You should work with your physician to establish SMBG goals that are right for you.

ADA General Guidelines for Average Target Blood Glucose Levels

Test Time	Whole Blood Meter Value	Plasma Meter Value
Preprandial (fasting or before meals)	80–120 mg/dl (4.4–6.7 mmol/l)	90–130 mg/dl (5–7.2 mmol/l)
At bedtime	100–140 mg/dl (5.6–7.8 mmol/l)	110–150 mg/dl (6.1–8.3 mmol/l)
Two hours postprandial (after meals)	under 140 mg/dl (7.8 mmol/l)	under 160 mg/dl (8.9 mmol/l)

The Monitor and Other Equipment

Your first order of business is choosing a monitor that's accurate, easy to use, and comfortable. In some cases, your insurance plan may dictate the brand or type you get. If you do have some latitude in selecting a meter, be sure to ask for recommendations. Your diabetes educator, members of your support group, and physician are all good sources.

The U.S. FDA regulations for the manufacture of blood glucose monitors suggest that monitors be accurate within 20 percent of laboratory reference values. That may seem like a lot, but as long as your meter is consistent in its readings and you know how much it differs from laboratory values (which your doctor can help you determine), the variance isn't too critical. If a reading seems excessively high or low, try testing again.

Anatomy of a Meter

Blood glucose monitors come in all shapes and sizes, but there are some common features that most share:

- **Display.** Blood glucose readings are digitally displayed on a small screen in either whole blood or plasma equivalent results. Both test the amount of glucose in whole blood, but "plasma equivalent" meters run the results through an extra mathematical formula that displays what the amount of glucose in just the plasma (the fluid in which red and white blood cells are suspended) should be. Because blood glucose tests performed in a laboratory use plasma results, some people find this a convenient feature for comparison purposes. It's important to know what type of numbers your meter is using, since plasma equivalents run approximately 12 to 15 percent higher than whole-blood results.
- **Buttons and beepers.** The operator's manual for your monitor will explain the button functions. Your meter may also have special audio signals to let you know when a test is complete or alert you to highs and lows.
- **Test strip slot.** Your blood sample goes on a test strip, which is inserted into the meter. Some meters use self-enclosed test strip drums or cartridges, which are automatically fed into the meter and don't require any user handling.
- **Memory.** Most modern meters have some type of memory feature that can record a predetermined number of glucose readings. Some will also let you mark readings taken around insulin doses and generate different average glucose readings.
- **Battery.** Meters are battery powered, and many have a warning system that will tell you when the battery power starts to get low.

Other bells and whistles you may find on your glucose monitor include large displays or voice modules for patients with vision problems, backlit displays or glow-in-the-dark cases for easy night testing, and computer compatibility for downloading glucose data to special software programs.

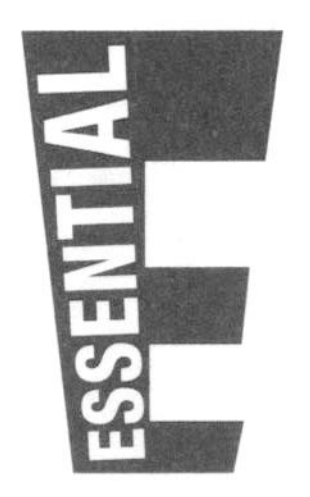

Bring your blood glucose meter along to your doctor's appointments. If you're new to testing, or you're using a new brand of meter, your physician can compare the readings with laboratory values to ensure accuracy. In addition, your doctor may also want to see your technique when you review your self-management.

Moreover, there are a growing number of meters on the market that do more than just test blood glucose levels. The InDuo (LifeScan/Novo Nordisk) is a glucose monitor and an insulin delivery system. The Precision Xtra (MediSense) tests both blood glucose and blood ketone levels. The BD Latitude (Becton, Dickinson, and Company) is an integrated meter, insulin pen case, and supply organizer. These multitasking meters may be a good choice for you if you have type 1 diabetes and want to cut down on your clutter.

Obtaining the Blood Sample

You draw the blood for testing with a lancet, which is a small, fine needle. Lancets come in a small plastic case and can be used alone or inserted into a spring-loaded lancing device, which quickly pierces the skin at a preset depth.

Lancets are available in different gauges (e.g., 21 gauge, 30 gauge)—the higher the gauge, the narrower the lancet, and the smaller the insertion hole at the test site. A higher-gauge lancet will, theoretically, make for a less painful stick (although factors such as skin sensitivity and test site factor in, too). High-gauge lancets may also be preferable for children.

Many monitors come with a separate lancing pen, while others have a lancing device integrated into the monitor itself. Lancing devices can also be purchased separately. Because each use damages the needle slightly and makes subsequent tests more painful, it's recommended that a fresh lancet be loaded with each test. If you must reuse a lancet, clean it thoroughly with alcohol first, and never use someone else's used lancet.

The lancets you use depend on three factors:

1. The requirements of the meter
2. The sensitivity and condition of your fingers (for instance, calloused fingers may require thicker lancets)
3. The size of the blood sample required—some meters only require a blood drop as small as a pinhead

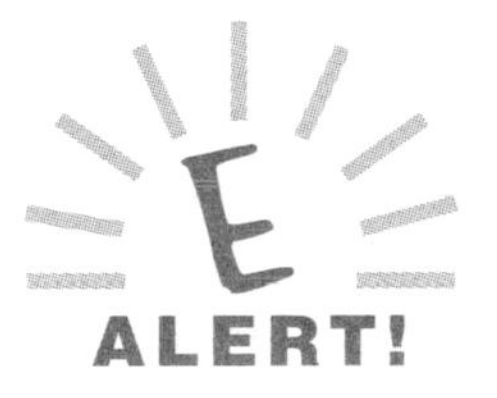

Each year, an estimated 600,000 to 800,000 Americans suffer needlestick injuries, often from improperly discarded syringes and other medical supplies. Lancets need to be disposed of in a puncture-proof container. Find out if your pharmacy has a "sharps bring back" program, and check with your municipality about procedures for medical waste disposal.

Alternative Site Testing

To the relief of sore fingers everywhere, there is a newer breed of glucose monitors available that allow testing on less sensitive parts of the body, such as the forearm or thigh. These alternative site meters may be a good choice for you if you have sensitive fingers and you find yourself testing infrequently because of it.

However, be aware that test results from alternative sites of the body can vary from fingertip testing. Blood from the fingertips may register glucose changes in the body faster than blood from other testing sites. The FDA has required alternative site meter manufacturers to label their products with this information. If you are experiencing signs of hypoglycemia, or if you have hypoglycemic unawareness, always test from your fingertips to ensure the most accurate readings.

Test Strips

A test strip is a small rectangular piece of chemically treated paper that collects your blood sample for analysis by your monitor. The accuracy of your blood tests depends on the quality and treatment of your test strips, so don't gamble with your health by cutting corners. Using expired strips is dangerous, because they may not be able to detect your glucose levels accurately. Test strips are costly, and buying strips in large quantities is usually cheaper than the smaller-quantity packages. However, if you find yourself ending up with half-used containers of strips and have to throw them away, you haven't saved anything.

Many third-party manufacturers (companies that manufacture strips compatible with other manufacturers' brands of meters) produce strips for use in a variety of meter makes and models. These third-party strips can often be less expensive than the brand name. However, you need to be sure that they have been tested for use with your specific monitor. The test strip package labeling and directions for use should list this information. If you don't see your monitor make and model listed, don't buy the strips. Your monitor manufacturer often can provide you with a list of compatible third-party test strips.

Always keep your test strips out of excessive heat and moisture. The bathroom is a poor choice for storage, as humidity can affect strip accuracy. Storing your strips inside of your meter case in their original package will ensure that they stay clean.

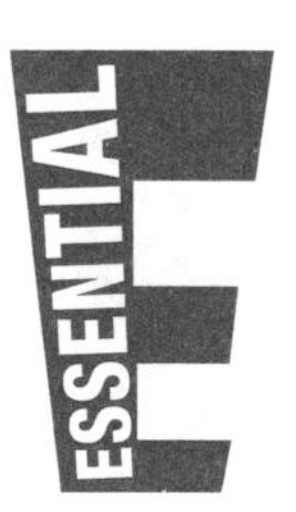

Extreme temperature swings can affect the accuracy of meters and test strips. For this reason, avoid stowing your meter and supplies in your car in hot or cold weather, and don't leave your equipment outside in direct sunlight or extreme cold.

Accessorize!

Stuffing your meter in a back pocket or letting it float around in the bottom of your purse with last year's ATM receipts, broken breath mints, and other assorted junk isn't a good idea. You trust your health to this piece of equipment, so treat it carefully. Many meters come with a carrying case for protection—use it. If yours didn't include a case, a well-padded cosmetic bag, shaving kit, or similar container will do the trick, too.

Your test strips and control solution also need to be kept clean, dry, and at room temperature. Keep them in the case with your monitor and lancing supplies, and you'll have everything properly stored and together when you need it.

How It Works

So how do you test? First, read the instructions. Even if you're a "do first, ask for directions later" kind of a person, stifle that instinct. Every meter operates a little differently, and there may be calibration or other steps required that are outlined in the directions for use.

Glucose testing involves using a lancet to prick your fingertip or other area of your body to get a blood sample. When performed on the finger, this is called a finger stick. The blood drop that comes out of the finger stick is then placed on a test strip that has been inserted into the glucose meter. (Many newer meters feature strips that actually draw in or absorb the blood sample.) Once the meter detects an adequate sample of blood on the strip, it will measure the amount of glucose present and display the results on the screen in either an mg/dl or mmol/l reading. Some meters will display readings that are excessively high or low with special alarms or warnings. Getting results can take anywhere from a few seconds to a minute.

Following are some tips to improve the ease, accuracy, and usefulness of your testing:

- Wash and rinse your hands thoroughly. Any food, medication residue, or other substances on your fingers can affect test results.
- If you use rubbing alcohol on the test site, let it dry before lancing. Pricking the skin before the alcohol dries can cause stinging or burning.
- Experiment with different gauge lancets. The thickness, or gauge, of your lancet affects both the size of the blood sample and how painful it feels.
- Experiment with different lancet depths. Spring-loaded lancing devices often offer an option for adjusting how far into the skin the needle pierces.

- Get the blood flowing to your hands before you stick yourself. If you have problems getting an adequate drop of blood, running your hands under warm water, rubbing them together, or shaking them at your sides can stimulate circulation.

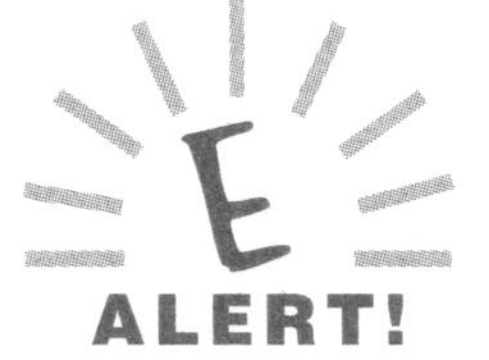

Always have a blood glucose monitor close at hand. Having several meters stored at the places where you spend most of your time—home, the office, school—will ensure that you can always test if an unexpected high or low hits. If you think you are experiencing a hypoglycemic episode but don't have a meter with you, take some fast-acting carbohydrates to bring glucose levels back up, then test as soon as possible.

Troubleshooting

Even with the most fastidious testing methods, sometimes the numbers just won't seem right. If you think your technique may be to blame, review the operator's manual and test again. Certain medical conditions (such as anemia) and substances (such as vitamin C) can influence glucose testing results. Talk with your doctor if you have coexisting medical conditions or are taking other medications or supplements outside of your diabetes drugs.

Quality Control

If your readings are off, you may be able to use quality-control tools that are part of your meter kit. Control solution is a glucose-based liquid that is used in place of blood to ensure your meter is working correctly. If the reading on your meter matches the range of values on the control solution label, your meter should be accurate. A special electronic control strip may also be included with the meter that is used to ensure it is operating properly. Read your meter instructions to find out more on how to use these features.

Calibration

Glucose monitors must be calibrated for use with your test strips before use. Test strips will be labeled with a number that must be entered into the meter. Check both your owner's manual and test strip documentation for information on calibrating test strip type. If your strips are calibrated correctly and the readings still seem to be off, try one from a new package (and report problems with the old package to the strip manufacturer).

Keep It Clean

A dirty meter or dirty, damaged test strips can give false readings. The instructions for use that came with your glucose monitor should tell you how and when to clean it. Be aware that some monitors are not designed to be cleaned, so always read the directions first.

Wear and Tear

Even the most rugged meters will wear out eventually. If you're getting frequent error codes or your monitor is giving erratic readings, it may just be time to trade in your trusty old friend for a newer model.

Tracking Your Test Results

Your test results are most useful if you view them in the context of the rest of your day. Log your readings, along with your medications, insulin, food intake, exercise, and other significant events. Over time, patterns will emerge, and you will probably discover certain triggers that make your blood glucose levels fluctuate. Your doctor can help you interpret the data even further.

Some glucose monitors have memory features that allow you to store several weeks' or even months' worth of readings, compute averages, and indicate which readings occurred in conjunction with an insulin shot. These can also be helpful in detecting patterns.

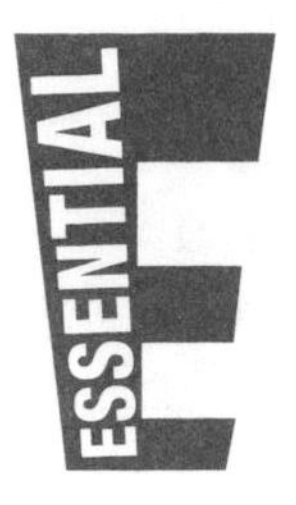

If a reading seems wrong, test again. If it still looks wrong and you feel as if your blood glucose is low, take a fast-acting carbohydrate until symptoms subside. When you're feeling better, call the customer service department for your meter manufacturer and run through any additional troubleshooting steps they offer.

Logbooks

Many monitors come with a logbook for recording the results, but a notebook will do the job just as well. When recording your readings, make sure you note the time of the test (i.e., preprandial/postprandial) and the time and amount of medication and/or insulin taken. For an even more complete picture of what's happening with your blood glucose levels, you can also note what you eat at each meal.

The sample logbook shown here includes entry spaces for "before meal" (preprandial) and "after meal" (postprandial) blood glucose results, plus a space to record the carbs consumed in each meal and the accompanying insulin dose or mixed dose (if applicable). There's also a space for bedtime and snack test readings. Finally, a comments area is available for notes on special circumstances that may have impacted your blood sugar that day, such as exercise, specific foods, and illness.

Logbooks come in many configurations, and may also include space for checking off oral medication doses, a record of food intake for each meal, and detailed info on daily exercise. Try out a few formats until you find one that works well for you.

Companion Software

An increasing number of meter manufacturers are putting out monitors with companion software that analyzes glucose readings both for patients and their doctors. This software can be an excellent tool for charting long-term progress of glucose control, especially if it has the ability to generate printable reports and charts, and to graph trends. You can also purchase third-party software to track and analyze your blood glucose readings.

Another new trend is the advent of blood glucose monitor modules that can be used with personal data assistants (PDAs) or Palm units. These have the added advantage of being integrated into a device that the user is already familiar with and keeps at hand. They can also easily save and analyze data.

Daily Diabetes Log

Week of: ______________

Day	Breakfast		Lunch		Dinner		Bedtime		Other/Snack		Comments
	Pre / Post	Carbs / Insulin	Pre / Post	Carbs / Insulin	Pre / Post	Carbs / Insulin	Pre / Post	Carbs / Insulin	Pre / Post	Carbs / Insulin	Diet, exercise, ketones, illness, stress
Mon		/		/		/		/		/	
Tue		/		/		/		/		/	
Wed		/		/		/		/		/	
Thu		/		/		/		/		/	
Fri		/		/		/		/		/	
Sat		/		/		/		/		/	
Sun		/		/		/		/		/	
Avg.											

▲ Always record your glucose readings, along with medication, food intake, and other important treatment notes.

Ways to Reduce the "Ouch" Factor

One of the biggest deterrents to frequent testing is the pain and soreness caused by finger sticks. Recently, the most significant and widely available innovation to help solve that problem is the alternative site monitor, which allows the patient to replace finger sticks with blood drawn in less sensitive areas of the body such as the forearm and thigh. These meters may require smaller blood samples than traditional models, but as previously discussed, the readings they give may vary from fingertip readings.

The only FDA-approved lancing device that does not use a traditional needle lancet is the Personal Lasette Plus (Cell Robotics). The Lasette uses a laser system to puncture the skin and draw blood from the finger, and is said to be no more painful than a quick snap from a rubber band. A doctor's prescription is needed to purchase the unit, which is approved for ages five and up. It's expensive (about $1,000), but along with reducing the pain of traditional lancets it also eliminates the problem of sharps disposal.

Trend Testing

As of early 2003, there are two FDA approved noninvasive monitoring devices currently on the U.S. market that are designed to supplement–but not to replace–regular self-monitoring of blood glucose. These products, the GlucoWatch G2 Biographer and the Medtronic MiniMed CGMS (continuous glucose-monitoring system), are useful for recording and identifying blood glucose trends over time. They also both require calibration with finger stick testing.

The GlucoWatch (Cygnus, Inc.) uses a low-frequency electrical current to painlessly draw out and measure glucose through the skin. The device, which displays readings on a watch interface at predetermined intervals, stores up to 8,500 glucose readings up to thirteen hours a day. Results can be downloaded into special software that compiles the data and graphs trends. The second-generation GlucoWatch, the G2, was introduced in the U.S. market in September 2002.

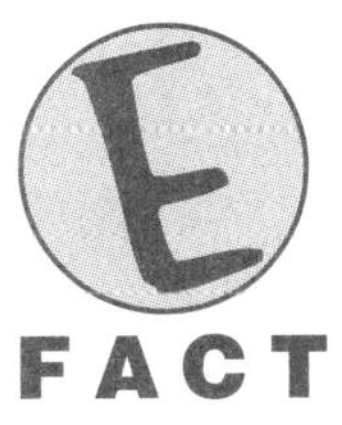

The GlucoWatch was found to be highly effective in predicting hypoglycemic episodes in several clinical studies, which is perhaps one of the biggest benefits of the monitor. The G2 allows you to set personal alarm levels for high and low readings, and is approved for use in adults and children ages seven and up.

The Medtronic MiniMed CGMS is an implantable device that measures glucose levels every five minutes for up to three days. It consists of a sensor, which is inserted under the skin by a physician, and a control module that stores the blood glucose data. The sensor reads glucose levels in cellular (interstitial) fluid. The CGMS does not display glucose readings on the module itself. After you've been on the system for three days, your physician can download the blood glucose data using special software and analyze the results.

On the Horizon

One continuous glucose-monitoring device currently under development by SpectRx measures glucose levels in interstitial fluid (ISF). The SpectRx device uses a laser to create microscopic holes through which the ISF is collected. The ISF is then measured in a sensor patch.

Another product, the Symphony (Sontra Medical Corporation), uses ultrasound to detect glucose levels. Insulin pump manufacturer Animas is also developing an implantable sensor that uses infrared spectroscopy to continuously measure glucose levels, which are then transmitted to a remote receiver. A third monitor still in the prototype stage, the SugarTrac (LifeTrac Systems), employs near infrared light to measure glucose concentration in the earlobe.

Hopefully, the further exploration of glucose monitoring technologies that reduce patient discomfort will increase testing compliance. In the meantime, if finger sticks have you avoiding your meter, a good alternative site monitor can help ease your pain.

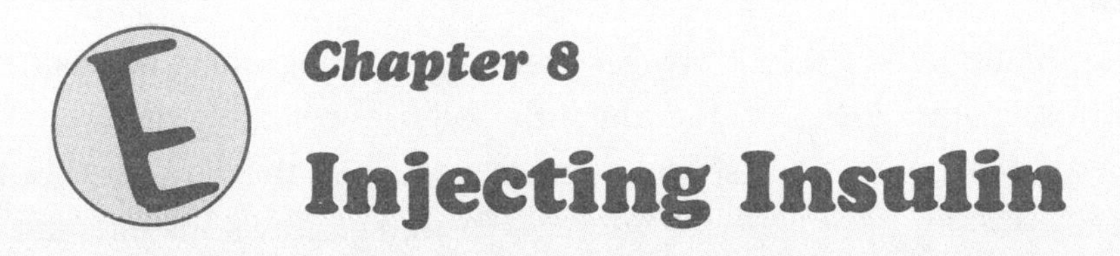

Chapter 8

Injecting Insulin

All people with type 1 diabetes require insulin injections to live, and many type 2 patients end up needing insulin to control their disease. Before the discovery of insulin in the 1920s, the only way to control type 1 diabetes was through a near-starvation diet, and patients consequently did not have a very long life span. Today, electronically programmed pumps can deliver precise doses of the life-saving hormone, and new noninvasive forms of delivering insulin are on the horizon.

How Does Injected Insulin Work?

Injected insulin mimics the action of the hormone produced by the body. Once it is injected under the skin and into the subcutaneous (below the skin) fat layer, it starts stimulating glucose uptake by both skeletal muscle and fat cells, while at the same time signaling the liver to slow or stop glucose production.

The first insulin, isolated by Sir Frederick Banting and Charles Best (with help from J.J.R. Macleod and J.B. Collip), was extracted from the pancreas of a cow. The first few decades of insulin therapy used both bovine (cow) and porcine (pig) derived insulin. Today's insulins are created in the laboratory, cultured from bacteria and yeast with a technology known as *recombinant DNA*.

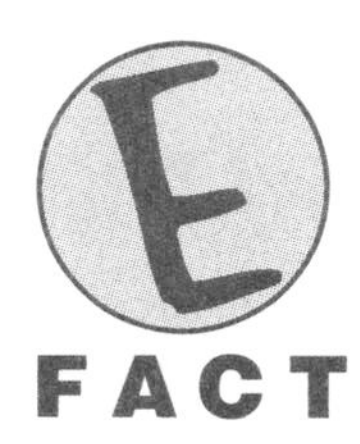

FACT

Manufacturers of animal-derived insulin have completely phased out bovine insulin from the American market and greatly reduced porcine insulin production. It is still possible to have beef and pork insulin imported into the United States for medical purposes.

Insulin Types and Quantities

Insulin comes in several different strengths and actions. A rapid-acting insulin such as Humalog is injected immediately before a meal and starts working in under fifteen minutes. Its peak of action (when it is working the hardest) is between sixty to ninety minutes after injection, about the time when blood sugar levels would be at their height after a meal. Regular insulin starts working thirty to sixty minutes after injection and peaks in three to five hours. NPH insulin is a longer-lasting insulin with a slower onset and peak action.

Insulin mixes can also be used to "cover" a meal; the most common premixed insulin is 70/30 (NPH and regular insulin). Newer long-acting insulins such as insulin glargine (Lantus) are designed to provide twenty-four-hour coverage. You and your doctor will choose an appropriate insulin or mix of insulins based on your particular blood glucose patterns.

Insulins by Type, Onset, Peak, and Duration

Type	*Onset*	*Peak*	*Duration*
Rapid-Acting			
Humalog (lispro)	<15 min.	30–90 min.	<5 hours
NovoLog (aspart)	10–20 min.	1–3 hours	3–5 hours
Regular (R)			
Humulin R	30–60 min.	2–3 hours	4–6 hours
Novolin R	30 min.	2.5–5 hours	8 hours
Velosulin BR	30 min.	1–3 hours	8 hours
NPH (N)			
Humulin N	2–4 hours	4–10 hours	14–18 hours
Novolin N	90 min.	4–12 hours	24 hours
Lente (L)			
Humulin L	3–4 hours	4–12 hours	16–20 hours
Novolin L	2.5 hours	7–15 hours	22 hours
Ultralente			
Humulin U	6–10 hours	minimal	20–30 hours
Premixed			
Humalog 75/25	15	1–6.5 hours	18–26 hours
Humulin 70/30	15–30 min.	2–12 hours	18–24 hours
Novolin 70/30	30 min.	2–12 hours	24 hours
Humulin 50/50	15–30 min.	2–12 hours	18–24 hours
Long-Acting Basal			
Lantus (glargine)	1.5 hours	none	24 hour

Compiled from Eli Lilly, Novo Nordisk, and Aventis product labeling information. These are general guidelines only. A number of factors can impact insulin action, including the injection site, time of day, and exercise.

The insulin premixes (i.e., 70/30, 75/25, 50/50) are convenient, commonly prescribed insulin combinations. They eliminate any operator error with trying to draw up two different insulin types, and are a boon to those people who may have vision problems or find mixing insulins difficult for other reasons.

Insulin Dosage

Your insulin dose will depend on the type and action of your insulin. Your doctor will tell you exactly what kind and how much insulin to inject, and when you should be taking it. However, the amount of regular insulin taken before meals will have to be calculated "on the fly" based on how many carbohydrates you are going to eat. You'll have to do a little bit of math to determine your dose.

The rule of thumb is that each unit of regular insulin covers about 15 grams of carbs (the insulin to carbohydrate ratio). For every 50 mg/dl blood sugar is above the target range, an additional unit of insulin should be added (the blood sugar to insulin ratio). So if you were planning on a dinner of 90 carbs and your blood sugar was 100 mg/dl over target, 8 units of insulin would be necessary (6 to cover the carbs and 2 for the blood sugar). However, the insulin to carb ratio is different for everyone, as is the insulin to blood sugar ratio, and you should work with your diabetes health care provider to track your glucose levels and determine what ratios are right for you.

Selecting the Delivery Device

Insulin must be injected into the subcutaneous layer of fat. As of early 2003, the only approved devices for administering insulin were syringes, insulin pens, and air-propelled injection devices. The type you choose will depend on your insulin prescription, budget, insurance coverage, and comfort level.

Choosing a Syringe

Syringes are probably the least expensive option, are readily available at virtually any pharmacy, and are easy to operate. If your insulin regimen requires mixing two types of insulins that aren't commonly available in a premixed pen, a syringe is your only choice.

Syringes come in a variety of sizes, from 30 to 100 units (from 1/33 of a cc to 1 cc). Some come with half-unit markings. When you're shopping for syringes, make sure you choose a type with markings that are easy for you to read and that accommodate your regular dosage.

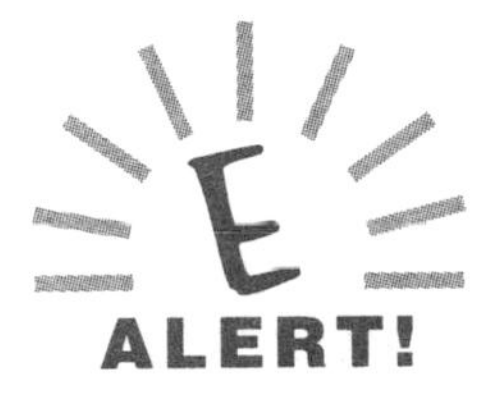

Overseas, insulin dilutions and measurements are a little different, with U-40 (40 units of active insulin in each milliliter of liquid) being the standard instead of U-100 (100 units of active insulin in each milliliter of liquid). If you're traveling abroad, be aware of this important difference.

Insulin Pens

Pens cost more but have the benefit of eliminating the step of drawing insulin from the vial. Instead, a pen uses a premeasured insulin cartridge, which usually contains either 150 or 300 units of insulin. Pens are either disposable, one-use models or reusable. The reusable ones allow you to insert and dispose of insulin cartridges, which you buy separately. Both types require the use of disposable pen needles, also purchased separately.

An insulin pen resembles just that, a pen. You uncap it to reveal the pen needle, then "dial up" your dose by turning the barrel until the correct number of units is displayed. After priming, you put the pen against the injection site and press a button to administer the insulin.

Other Injection Devices

Jet injection devices use air pressure to force insulin through the skin without actually puncturing it. They are more expensive than both pens and syringes, and can require more training to use effectively. The air pressure must be adjusted to propel the insulin strongly enough to penetrate the skin but lightly enough not to bruise. Finding a balance can take a little time.

For people who are deathly afraid of the needle, a jet injector may be a good choice. However, at prices ranging from $400 to $600, they require a significant initial investment (although eventually they will pay for themselves). Some people find them bulky to carry conveniently, as they are bigger than both syringes and pens.

Injecting Insulin

Once you have your delivery device selected, your prescription filled, and your resolve set, you're ready to give yourself a shot. Before you start, wash your hands thoroughly and examine the bottle of insulin. If you are injecting a clear insulin like lispro, you should look for crystals, cloudiness, or debris, and dispose of the bottle if you find any. For users of cloudy, long-acting insulins like Ultralente, you will have to gently mix the insulin in the vial by rolling it back and forth between your hands about twenty times. When the color appears even, it is mixed. Never shake the bottle, as this can damage the insulin.

You will also need three alcohol swabs, a syringe (or another device for injecting insulin), and a sharps disposal container.

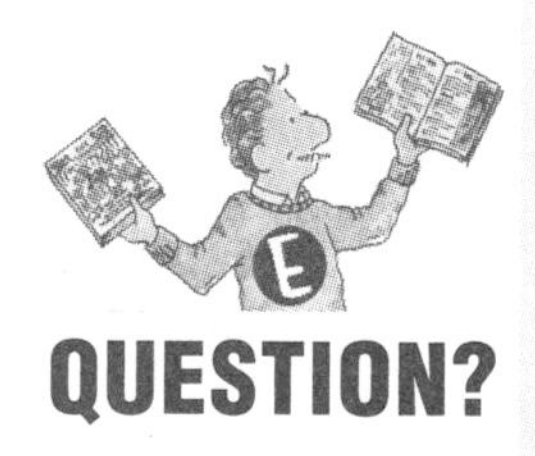

QUESTION?

My friend said that I could die if I injected an air bubble along with my insulin! Is that true?
Your friend was probably referring to air embolism, which can occur when air bubbles are injected into the circulatory system and block a blood vessel (this is not necessarily fatal). Since insulin is injected into the subcutaneous fat, this isn't a risk. But bubbles are bad for another reason—they throw off your dosing.

Drawing Up the Insulin

For those of you who use a pen, pump, or jet injector, drawing up insulin will not be an issue. Still, it's a good idea to know how to do it in case you are ever without your regular supplies and need to use a syringe. Your diabetes educator and/or doctor will go over this procedure as well. Here are the basic steps:

1. Open the insulin vial or bottle and mark the date on the label.
2. Wipe off the top of the insulin vial with an alcohol swab.

3. Uncap both the plunger and the needle of the syringe.
4. Draw in air to the syringe by pulling out the plunger until the stopper reaches the unit mark of what your insulin dose will be.
5. Push the syringe needle down through the rubber stopper in the insulin vial. Do *not* press down the plunger yet.
6. After the needle is all the way in, push the plunger all the way down to inject the air into the bottle.
7. Turn the syringe and bottle upside down. Make sure that the tip of the needle is still submerged in the insulin. If it isn't, pull the syringe out slightly until it is.
8. Slowly pull the syringe plunger out to draw the insulin until the stopper reaches the correct dosage mark.
9. Check for air bubbles. If there are some, push the insulin back in and redraw until none are visible.
10. Turn the bottle and syringe right-side up and carefully remove the syringe from the vial.

Choosing and Preparing a Site

Insulin should be injected into fat to do its job properly. This makes the fatty areas of the body—the butt, abdomen, thighs, and back of the upper arms—the most appropriate spots for giving injections. Don't choose your bicep, calf, or any other muscular area of your body. Muscle will accelerate the speed of your insulin action, and it hurts more to boot.

You can't inject yourself in the same spot every time. If you do, lumpy deposits of fat (lipohypertrophy) will form at the site and make injections increasingly difficult. These deposits also slow absorption of the insulin. Injection rotation doesn't require you to move from one side of the body to the other; moving over an inch or so will do the trick. However, you do need to have a method of keeping track of your rotation schedule.

Giving the Injection

Now the moment you've been waiting for—actually injecting the insulin. If you're like most people, you approach the first solo shot with trepidation and possible fear. Know that you can, and will, do it. Even the most squeamish, needle-fearing patients find that a little practice has them shoving in the syringe without a second thought.

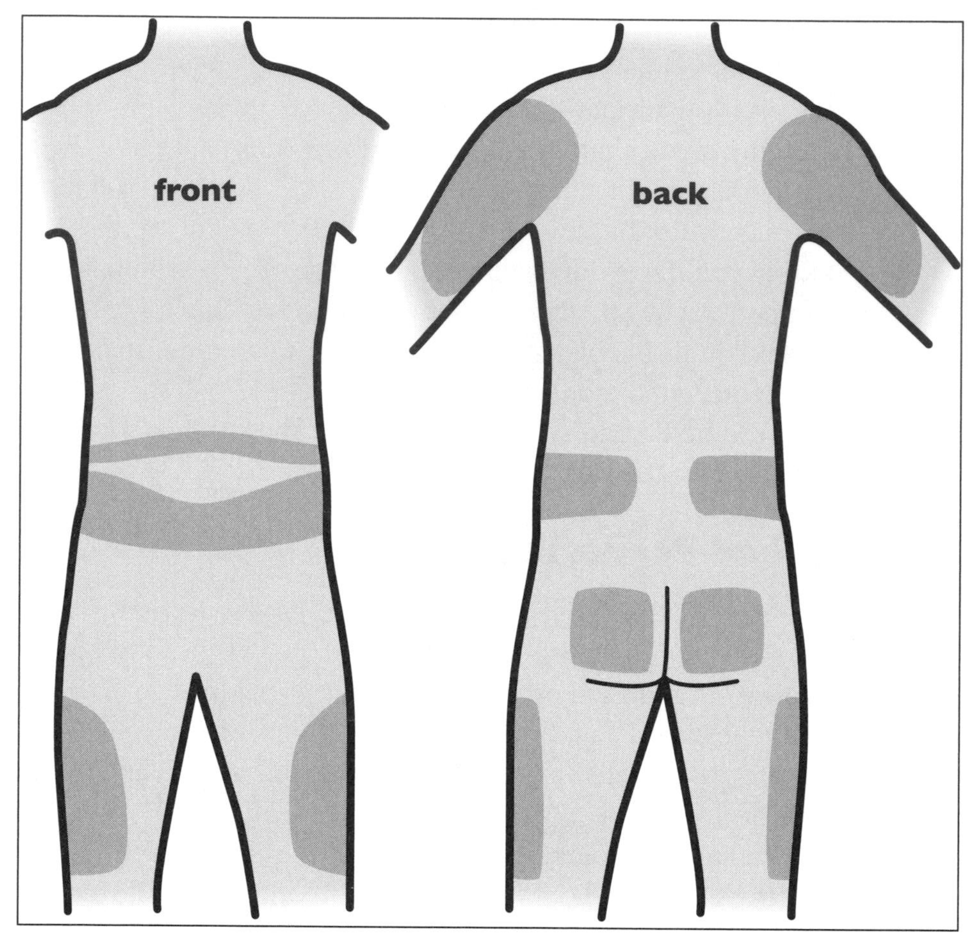

▲ **GOOD INJECTION SITES.** Once you have a spot picked out, clean it thoroughly with an alcohol swab to sterilize the area.

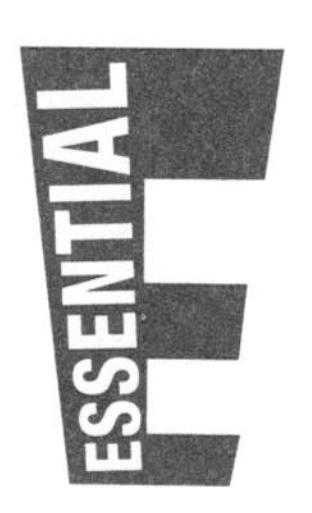

As for giving an injection with an insulin pen, the process is pretty much point and shoot after inserting the insulin cartridge and pen needle. Always read the manufacturer's directions completely for any procedures specific to the model or brand you use.

Your diabetes educator or doctor will teach you the proper method of finding a good injection site and giving yourself a shot. In fact, you may be given a syringe of saline in the office to "practice" your technique with. After you've chosen an appropriate site, follow these simple steps for giving yourself an almost painless syringe injection:

1. When you clean the area, let the alcohol dry completely before injecting to avoid a nasty sting.
2. Grab a roll of fat (or flesh) between your thumb and forefinger with your nonshooting hand. You do *not* want to inject into muscle, so choose appropriately.
3. Assess the area where you're injecting. If it's a fairly fatty site, you can use a 90-degree angle. Otherwise, you may have to try up to a 45-degree angle to avoid hitting muscle or blood vessels.
4. Hold the syringe like a dart, paper airplane, or anything else you'd want to sail through the air. Keep your thumb off the plunger until it's in.
5. The key to pain-free injection is to stick the needle in completely and quickly. One caution: If you're giving insulin to a child, start a little slower. It may take some experimentation to find the speed that is least painful.
6. Depress the plunger with your thumb slowly and steadily. As you get accustomed to the "feel," adjust your speed as needed.
7. Count to five before you pull out to avoid insulin leakage. Then pull out the syringe, let go of the site, and gently press against the site with an alcohol swab momentarily. You're done!

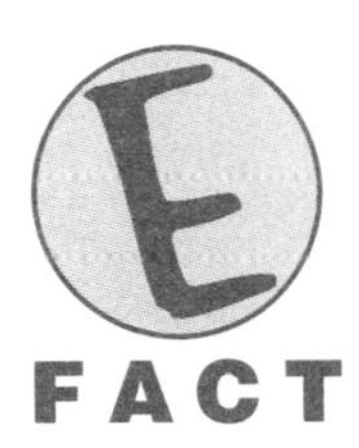

FACT

Oral, transdermal (patch), and inhaled insulin may some day be pain-free treatment options for U.S. diabetes patients. Oral insulin, which is delivered in a spray, has shown the most promise of the three technologies in clinical trials, as the lining of the mouth best absorbs the insulin.

Storing and Transporting Insulin

Hot or subzero cars, beach bags, or other extreme conditions can quickly deplete insulin's potency. If you're going to be traveling or participating in a recreational activity that will expose your insulin to the elements, be sure to have an insulated case that can keep it safe.

Some insulin manufacturers recommend refrigerated storage of their products; others can be stored at room temperature. Always read the insulin labeling and/or manufacturer's directions for use to find out exactly what storage requirements your particular insulin has.

When Good Insulin Goes Bad

You can tell a lot about insulin by just looking at it. Always check the expiration date of your insulin before you draw it up. Then take a moment to inspect the bottle. Rapid- and short-acting insulin should be clear, while intermediate- and long-acting insulin should look cloudy. The exception to the rule is glargine (Lantus), which is long-acting but is also clear. If your insulin has any crystals or debris in it, or looks cloudy when it should be clear, it could be either expired or spoiled. Never take a chance if it looks questionable; when it doubt, throw it out.

Of course, if you purchase insulin in prefilled pens, a visual inspection is impossible. Make sure to check expiration dates and handle and store pens properly, and you shouldn't have any issues.

Once you open a vial of insulin, its days are numbered, no matter what the expiration date. Typically, open insulin has a thirty-day shelf life. Always read the manufacturer's directions for use to find out how long a particular type of insulin will last after it has been opened.

All about Insulin Pumps

An insulin pump is a small external device about the size of a pager or cassette tape that is programmed to deliver a slow, continuous infusion (basal dose) of short-acting insulin into the body. At meal times, the wearer programs a bolus dose to cover the carbohydrates in the food she is going to eat.

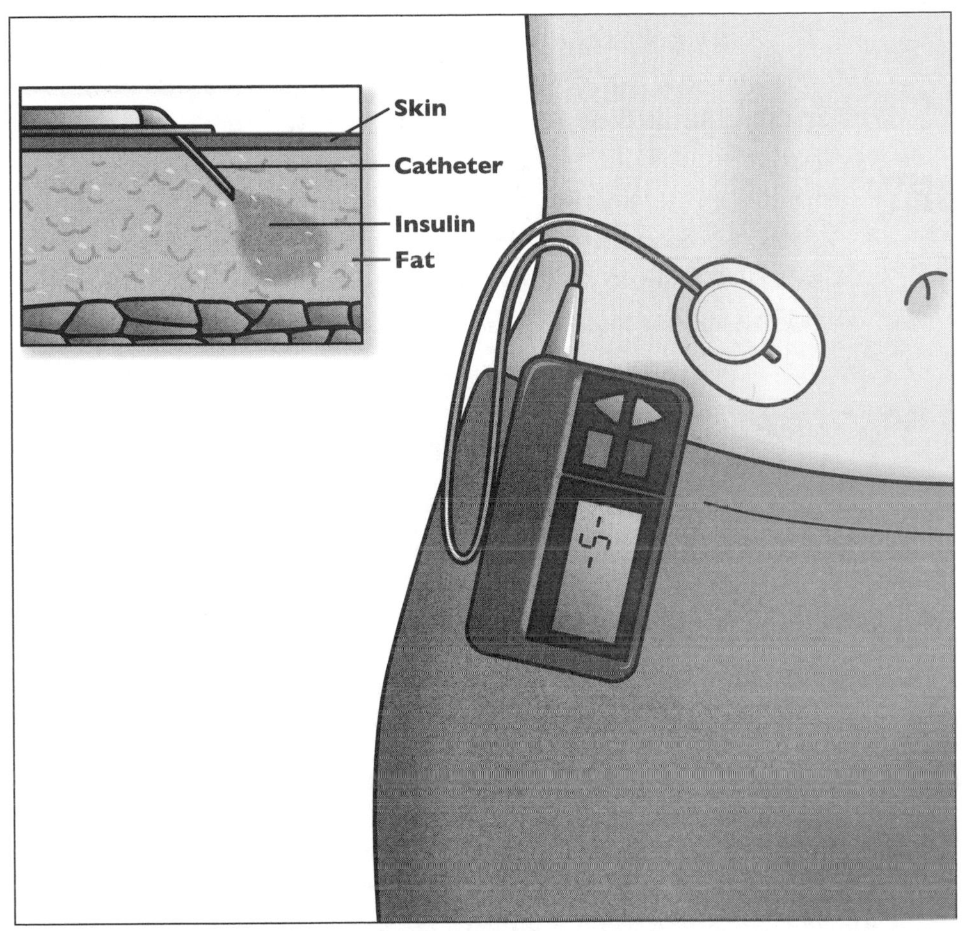

▲ An insulin pump administers insulin through a catheter in the abdominal fat to help control a person's blood sugar levels.

The pump itself consists of a reservoir for holding insulin, a digital display with dose and time information, and a port where the insulin leaves the unit. A piece of plastic tubing called an infusion set hooks on to the pump and carries the insulin from the unit to the body. A flexible plastic cannula or a needle is inserted just under the skin to deliver the insulin. Infusion sets must be changed every two to three days, and insertion sites rotated. Most people use the abdomen for insertion, although the same sites that can be used for insulin injection with a syringe can also be used for insertion.

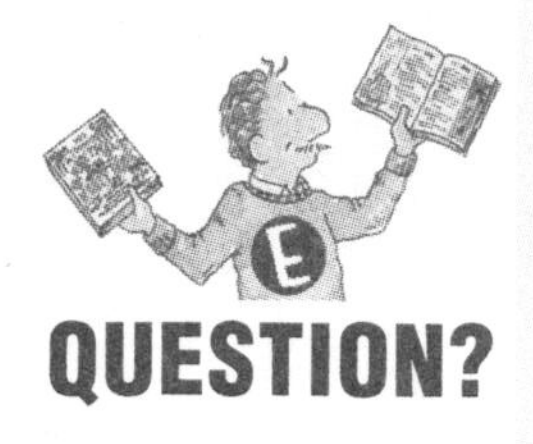

What are basal and bolus doses?
A basal dose is a slow, continuous infusion of small amounts of insulin that is designed to mimic the insulin secretion of a healthy pancreas. A bolus is a bigger dose of insulin taken before a meal to cover the resulting rise in blood glucose levels. Basal dosing should not be confused with basal insulin (i.e., Lantus), which is taken in a single dose but has continuous, twenty-four-hour nonpeaking action.

Who Pumps?

Children who crave added flexibility may be helped by a pump. People with "brittle" diabetes may find the pump helpful as well, because they can't get a handle on large glucose swings. People who suffer from nighttime lows (and accompanying morning highs) may also find that the pump helps them improve control; pumps can be programmed to increase their basal dose as morning glucose levels start to rise (i.e., the dawn phenomenon).

An insulin pump requires a dedicated patient—or, in the case of a small child, a dedicated parent. It is not a "plug and play" solution to your diabetes. Blood glucose levels must still be tested at least four times daily, bolus doses for meals have to be computed and programmed, and infusion sets have to be changed regularly. But people who are willing and able to put in the effort often find that the pump gives them that elusive control that injections couldn't.

Practical Matters

Of course, being hooked up to a pump 24/7 does bring up all sorts of daily dilemmas. Following are a few pointers on pumps that may answer the more practical questions you may be asking yourself about pump therapy:

- *Many pumps are waterproof, or at the very least water-resistant.* So if you accidentally get them wet, you're covered. There are also a variety of special waterproof and shock-resistant cases available.

- *Infusion sets come with tubing that is several feet in length.* The extra length, which doesn't have to be used, comes in handy if you like to put your pump next to your bed at night, or even leave it out of the tub while you bathe or shower.
- *Pumps are worn to bed.* Pumps keep working even when you're sleeping. Good places for your pump to stay at night are under the pillow, in a pajama pocket, or on the nightstand.
- *Pumps can be discrete.* If you don't feel comfortable wearing your pump like a beeper, there are many alternatives. Special pouches and straps are also available to wear pumps on the body under clothing.
- *Pumps can be disconnected, usually up to an hour.* If you prefer to shower, swim, or have sex without the constant companionship of your pump, you can. Always check blood glucose levels when you hook back up.

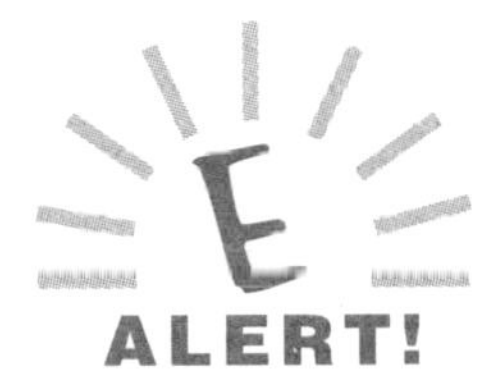

Be sure to read the directions for use for your particular pump thoroughly to find out its full range of capabilities. Your doctor may also have special instructions regarding pump disconnection and other issues.

Insurance and Medicare Issues

An insulin pump is a major investment. Pumps run around $5,000 (some higher, some lower), plus the costs of infusion sets and other supplies. The good news is that because tight control of glucose levels has been proved to reduce diabetes-related complications (in the DCCT and other trials), many insurance companies are more than willing to cover the price of a pump early, rather than pay the price of more expensive treatment for serious complications later.

Medicare will cover insulin pumps for both type 1 and type 2 diabetes patients, but they must meet strict clinical criteria to qualify. If you and your doctor think that you are a good candidate for the pump, work with him and his insurance coordinator to see if you meet Medicare guidelines.

Sharps Disposal

Insulin treatment with any form of sharps produces a lot of medical waste over time. It's important to dispose of needles and lancets properly to prevent injury to other people in your household and to anyone who comes in contact with your trash after it leaves the house.

Talk to the pharmacist where you purchase your syringes or diabetes supplies and find out if they offer a sharps bring-back or disposal program. These programs keep used sharps out of municipal landfills and incinerators where they have the potential to cause injury to workers.

If you don't have access to a sharps return program, there are many household products that come in containers ideal for sharps disposal. The main requirements are a puncture-resistant, unbreakable material and an opening that can be easily and tightly sealed. Liquid laundry detergent bottles, shampoo bottles, and coffee cans (with a hole for insertion) are all possibilities.

Label your sharps container "Used Medical Sharps—Do Not Recycle" with a waterproof marker so everyone who comes in contact with it will handle it appropriately.

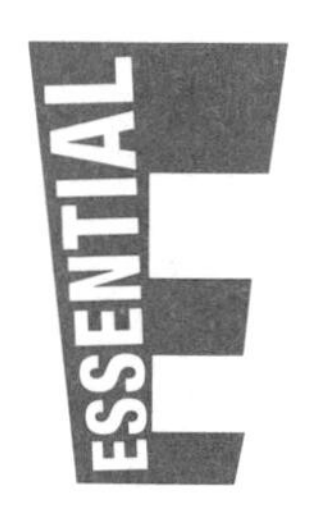

When you go on vacation, purchase a compact sharps disposal container for the trip. Another alternative is to use a small puncture-proof case, like a pencil box or an old thermos, until you return home and can dispose of sharps properly.

Never try to bend or recap a needle or lancet after you've used it. You can clip a needle with specially designed safety devices for this purpose, but never try to cut a needle with scissors or a knife. Instead, put your sharps directly into your disposal container.

When your container is full, put the top on tightly and seal it completely with heavy-duty tape. Find out if your municipality has a separate procedure for medical waste and follow the guidelines they provide. If your sharps container is to be put in with the regular trash pickup, make sure it goes in the garbage can and not the recycling bin.

Chapter 9

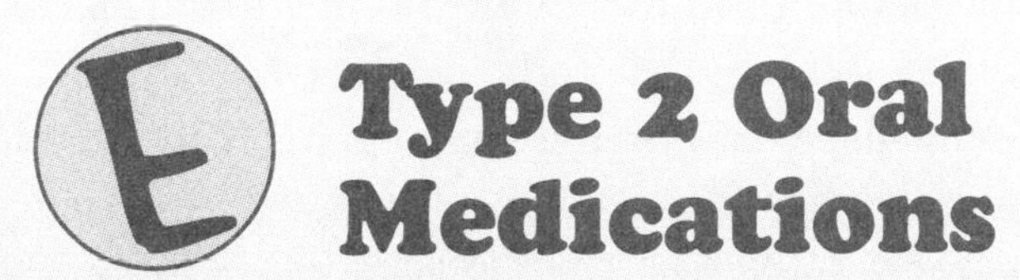

Type 2 Oral Medications

If you have type 2 diabetes, you may not need to rely on regular insulin injections, but there are times when despite all your best efforts and strict adherence to diet and regular exercise, your blood glucose levels just won't stay down. According to the CDC, only an estimated 17 percent of American adults control their type 2 diabetes with diet and exercise alone. The next line of defense is medication.

The Basics

If you're having trouble managing your type 2 diabetes with diet and exercise alone, your doctor may prescribe an oral medication to improve your blood glucose control. Some people with type 2 diabetes may also require insulin at some point, but oral medications are almost always given an adequate trial before moving on to insulin. Sometimes insulin therapy will be combined with an oral medication.

There are five main classes of oral medications for type 2 diabetes—sulfonylureas, biguanides, thiazolidinediones (also called TZDs or glitizones), alpha-glucosidase inhibitors, and meglitinides. Combination drugs, which combine medications across two classes of drugs, are also prescribed. Diabetes drugs that are currently on the U.S. market work in one of several ways:

- Inhibiting glucose production (biguanides, TZDs)
- Increasing insulin sensitivity (TZDs, some sulfonylureas)
- Stimulating insulin production (sulfonylureas, meglitinides)
- Blocking or slowing the digestion of carbohydrates (alpha-glucosidase inhibitors)
- A combination of two or more of the above actions (combination drugs)

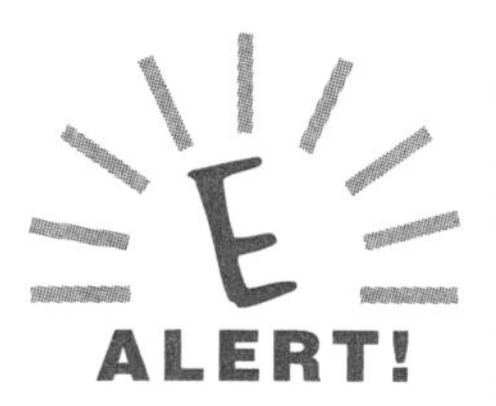

Make sure that your doctor is aware of all other medications—prescription, over-the-counter, or herbal—that you are taking. The therapeutic action of your diabetes drug may be either increased or reversed when taken with certain substances and medicines.

A Smooth Start

When you start on a new medication, log both the amount and timing of the dosage in your blood glucose logbook. This will give you and your health care provider a good idea of the impact the drug is having, and will allow her to make any necessary adjustments. You should note any side effects you have from the drug as well. Side effects will often wane and even disappear completely as your body becomes accustomed to the medication. In some cases, however, a dosage or medication change may eventually be required.

Your doctor should explain both the amount and frequency of your dose and any specific instructions about when to take it. However, it's also a good idea to read the drug labeling and directions for use that your pharmacist provides to ensure that you're taking your medication at the appropriate time and dosage. If the printed instructions seem to vary from what you have been told, call your physician immediately for instructions.

Practical Matters

Medication won't work if you forget to take it, so put your meds in a place where they are in sight and on your mind. If you take several prescription drugs, a medication organizer may be a good investment for you. There are many on the market, ranging from simple plastic caddies to more elaborate electronic systems. A watch with an audible alarm can also help keep you on track. Some people find keeping their medication with their blood glucose testing supplies convenient.

If you're prescribed a drug that must be taken with meals, keep it on the kitchen table or counter. You should also carry several pills in your purse, car, or another "always with you" spot for meals on the road. Make sure you rotate your extras weekly so they don't expire.

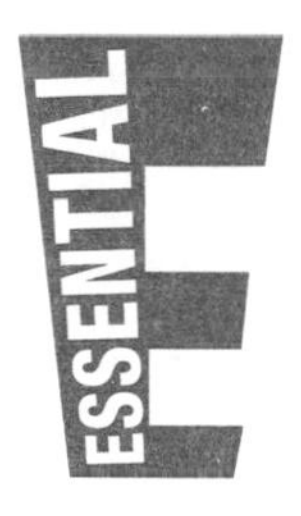

If your prescription is pricey, ask if a generic version is available. There are also a number of patient assistance programs available through drug manufacturers for people who can't afford their diabetes medications. See Appendix A for more resources.

Keeping meds within arm's reach can be hazardous in households with small children. Try keeping an empty pill bottle on the table as your reminder, and stow away the full bottle in a childproof cabinet.

Finally, always avoid storing your medications in heat, humidity, or direct sunlight, as temperature extremes can cause some drugs to lose their potency. And never take a drug that is past its expiration date.

Sulfonylureas

Sulfonylureas are the oldest class of oral diabetes medication, and were first introduced in the 1950s. Brand names of these drugs include Amaryl (glimepiride), DiaBeta (glyburide), Diabinese (chlorpropamide), Dymelor (acetohexamide), Glucotrol (glipizide), Glucotrol XL (glipizide), Glynase PresTab (glyburide), Micronase (glyburide), Orinase (tolbutamide), and Tolinase (tolazamide).

The oldest sulfonylurea drugs—Diabinese, Orinase, and Tolinase—require the largest dosage sizes (with daily doses ranging from 100 to 3,000 milligrams). The newer, or second-generation, sulfonylureas are much more potent and are typically prescribed at daily dosages ranging from just 1 to 40 milligrams. The newer drugs are usually taken twice daily before meals, except for Glucotrol XL and Glynase, which are extended-release medications that only need to be taken once daily. Your doctor will tell you when and how often to take your medication. Whatever the schedule, you should always try to take it consistently at the same time from day to day.

How They Work

Called "hypoglycemic agents," sulfonylurea drugs work by causing the pancreas to release more insulin, which in turn lowers blood glucose levels. For this reason, sulfonylureas may not be effective in people with long-standing diabetes who have lost most pancreatic beta cell function.

Amaryl (glimepiride), the newest of the sulfonylurea drugs, also works to decrease insulin resistance by binding with insulin receptors. So in addition to increasing insulin output, this drug also allows the body to more effectively use the insulin it produces.

Possible Side Effects

The most serious potential side effect of the sulfonylurea drugs is a hypoglycemic reaction, or low blood sugar episode. The older sulfonylureas, in particular, are more likely to cause this reaction if they are taken in conjunction with other medications.

There is some inconclusive clinical evidence that patients taking Orinase may run an increased chance of cardiovascular problems, so anyone with a history of heart problems should speak with his or her doctor about the potential risks.

Other possible side effects include, but are not limited to the following:

- Nausea
- Rash and/or itching
- Photosensitivity (sensitivity to sunlight)
- Dizziness
- Drowsiness
- Headache
- Weight gain

The potential for weight gain can be a problem for overweight patients, as weight gain will work against the benefits of the drug by increasing insulin resistance. Your physician may prefer to use a newer class of drugs, such as biguanides, for your treatment if you are significantly overweight.

Sulfonylureas (particularly chlorpropamide) also have the potential to react with alcohol, causing nausea, vomiting, and facial flushing. Talk to your doctor about this side effect before starting your prescription.

Biguanides

The biguanide class of drugs—Glucophage (metformin) and Glucophage XR (metformin hydrochloride, extended release)—is one of the most widely prescribed for type 2 diabetes. Biguanides are often preferred over sulfonylureas because they don't cause hypoglycemia nor do they promote weight gain. They have also been shown to have a positive effect on blood lipid levels.

Metformin is usually taken two to three times daily with meals. The extended release version is designed for once-a-day use, usually with an evening meal. It may also be used in conjunction with a sulfonylurea drug (Glucovance is metformin and glyburide) or with insulin therapy.

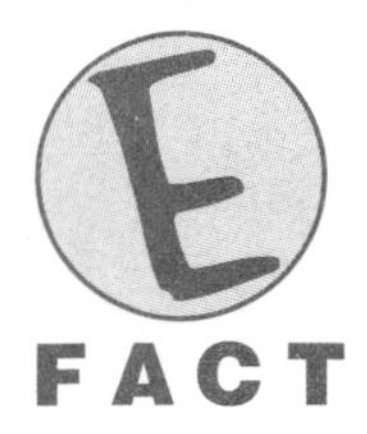
FACT

A 2002 study at the Hospital for Sick Children and the University of Toronto found that treatment with metformin lowered HbA1c levels and decreased the need for insulin in teens with type 1 diabetes who were considered to be in poor control of their diabetes.

How They Work

Metformin works by suppressing the amount of glucose your liver pumps out. It promotes weight loss and an improved cholesterol profile, which can reduce your insulin resistance. The United Kingdom Prospective Diabetes Study (UKPDS), a landmark twenty-year clinical study, found that overweight patients treated with metformin experienced a significantly lower mortality rate than those treated with sulfonylurea drugs and had a marked reduction in strokes and heart attacks.

Possible Side Effects

Metformin is not recommended for people with kidney or liver problems due to the risk of lactic acidosis, a rare but potentially fatal buildup of lactic acid in the bloodstream that occurs when the liver and kidneys do not adequately remove lactic acid. Signs of lactic acidosis include weakness, fatigue, dizziness, breathing problems, and unexplained muscle and/or stomach pain. If you experience any of these symptoms while taking metformin, seek prompt medical attention.

Biguanides are also not recommended for use in patients with congestive heart failure. Other potential side effects of metformin include:

- Gastrointestinal distress (gas and diarrhea)
- Nausea
- Metallic taste in the mouth
- Depletion of vitamin B_{12} levels

Because up to 30 percent of patients prescribed metformin experience gastrointestinal discomfort, dosage is generally started quite low and slowly increased.

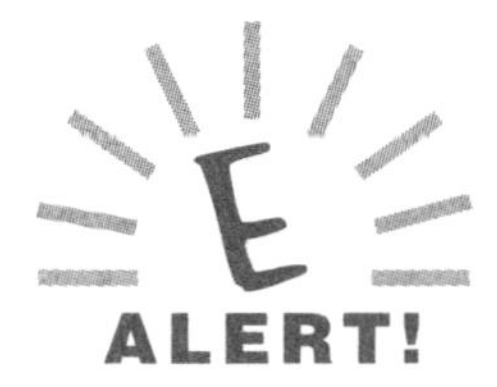

If you are undergoing any radiographic (i.e., x-ray or CT scan) procedure that involves injection of a contrast medium (i.e., dye) that contains iodine, you should stop taking metformin temporarily because of the increased risk of lactic acidosis. Metformin can be started again if kidney function is normal when it is reassessed forty-eight hours after the injection.

Thiazolidinediones (TZDs)

Actos (pioglitazone) and Avandia (rosiglitazone) are the two TZD drugs currently available in the United States. A third drug in the class, Rezulin (troglitazone), was withdrawn from the market in 2000 after reports of fatalities due to liver damage.

The FDA has approved Actos for use with insulin, metformin, or sulfonylureas. Avandia is cleared for use with metformin or sulfonylureas. Actos is usually taken once daily, and Avandia may be taken once or twice daily. Both can be taken with or without food.

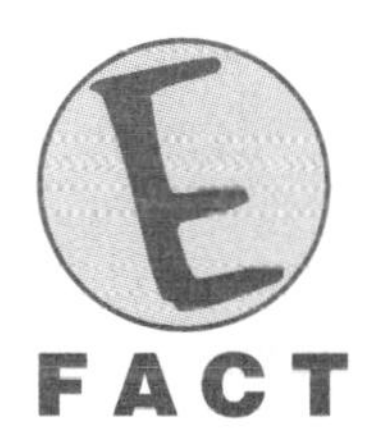

If you take birth control pills, TZD drugs can make them less effective. They can also increase fertility in women with polycystic ovary disease (PCOS). Women who take TZD drugs should speak with their doctor about contraceptive options.

How They Work

The TZD drugs, which are also called glitazones or insulin sensitizers, target the insulin receptors in muscle and fat cells to increase the level of insulin sensitivity in the body. They also reduce glucose production slightly, and can be effective in lowering blood pressure and triglyceride levels, and in increasing HDL (or "good") cholesterol. Because they lower glucose so effectively, they also reduce hyperinsulinemia (excess circulating insulin).

Possible Side Effects

Because of the associations found between Rezulin and liver failure, the FDA has imposed strict guidelines on assessing liver function in patients taking other TZD drugs. If you take a TZD, you must have regular testing of the liver enzyme ALT. ALT levels should be tested before treatment starts, every two months for the first year you take the drug, and as recommended by your doctor thereafter. Avandia or Actos should be discontinued if ALT levels rise more than three times the normal upper limit, and should not be started in patients who have ALT levels that are greater than 2.5 times higher than the normal upper limit.

Other side effects of TZD therapy may include:

- Edema (water retention) of the ankles or legs
- Anemia
- Weight gain
- Muscle weakness
- Headaches
- Fatigue
- Coldlike symptoms

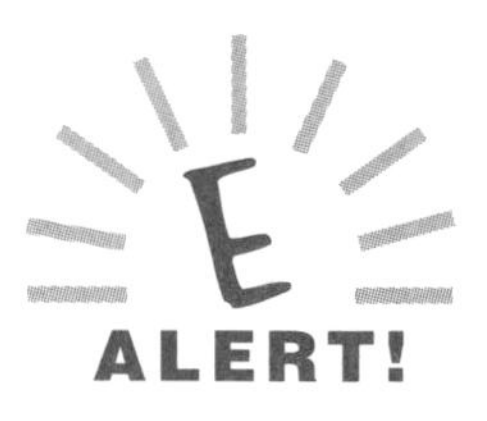

If a blood sugar low occurs when Glyset or Precose is taken in conjunction with a sulfonylurea or insulin, it should *not* be treated with fructose or sucrose (since AG inhibitors cause a slower digestion of these sugars). Instead, glucose gel or tablets, or milk (which contains lactose), should be used to boost blood glucose levels.

Alpha-Glucosidase Inhibitors (AG)

The alpha-glucosidase inhibitor class of type 2 drugs consists of Glyset (miglitol) and Precose (acarbose). Also called “starch blockers,” these medications must be taken at each meal with the first bite of food in order to be effective. AG inhibitors may be prescribed along with a sulfonylurea drug, metformin, or insulin for some patients.

How They Work

Glyset and Precose work by slowing digestion. More specifically, they block the enzymes responsible for the breakdown of carbohydrates in the intestine, so blood glucose rise is slower and steadier. They may be prescribed for you if you have a hard time keeping your postprandial (after meal) blood glucose levels under control. AG inhibitors may be a preferred therapy in overweight patients, since they do not promote weight gain like the sulfonylureas and TZDs do.

Possible Side Effects

Because of the way they work, most of the side effects of the AG inhibitors are gastrointestinal, and include bloating, diarrhea, gas, and cramping. However, like metformin, the uncomfortable side effects can be greatly reduced by starting with a small dose and gradually increasing it.

People with serious gastrointestinal disorders, including intestinal disease or obstructions, inflammatory bowel disease, and colonic ulceration, should not take AG inhibitors.

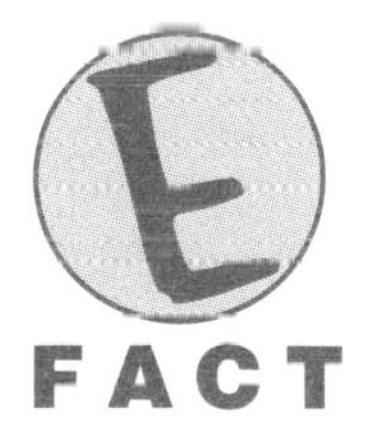

FACT

If you take oral medications for your type 2 diabetes and want to become pregnant, make an appointment to discuss your options with your doctor. None of the currently available oral medications are considered safe for use in pregnancy, but insulin is. Your doctor will probably suggest a switch to insulin before you start trying to conceive so you can stabilize your blood sugars on the new therapy.

Meglitinides

Prandin (repaglinide) and Starlix (nateglinide) are currently the only FDA-approved meglitinide class drugs in the United States. Like AG inhibitors, they are taken at meal times (usually about fifteen minutes before eating) to prevent a postprandial blood sugar rise. People who tend to test high after meals may benefit from treatment with meglitinide drugs.

Prandin is also FDA approved for use with the insulin sensitizers Actos (pioglitazone) and Avandia (rosiglitazone) and for use with metformin. Starlix is cleared for use with metformin.

How They Work

Meglitinides are short-acting oral hypoglycemic agents that bind to and stimulate the insulin-producing beta cells of the pancreas in response to the level of glucose in the bloodstream.

Taken before a meal, meglitinides can boost what is known as *first-phase insulin release,* the production of insulin that is a response to the initial boost of carb-generated blood glucose after a meal. Both Prandin and Starlix can be taken anywhere from right before up to thirty minutes prior to a meal.

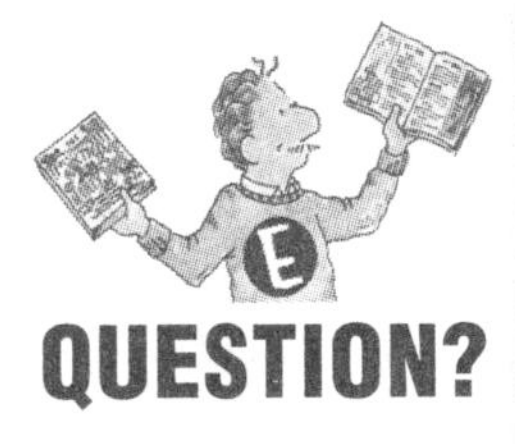

If I skip a meal, should I still take my meds?
First of all, try not to skip meals, as it's hard on blood glucose control. That said, it depends on the type of medication you take and the schedule you take it on. If you take an AG inhibitor or a meglitinide, you should skip the dose and take the next one with your next meal. As always, talk to your doctor about your specific situation.

Possible Side Effects

Hypoglycemia can occur as a side effect of the meglitinide drugs. Symptoms of a low blood glucose episode include sweating, shakiness, dizziness, increased appetite, disorientation, heart palpitations, nausea, fatigue, and weakness. A hypo should be treated immediately with a fast-acting carbohydrate.

Patients new to type 2 medications may also experience weight gain with meglitinides. The most commonly reported side effects occurring with meglitinide drugs are:

- Cold and flu symptoms
- Headache

- Diarrhea and other gastrointestinal complaints
- Joint and back pain

If you take a meglitinide drug, you should monitor your blood glucose levels one hour and two hours after eating to ensure your medication is working properly. If blood sugar readings still seem too high, talk to your doctor about adjusting your dose.

Combination Drugs

Drugs that combine two classes of medications are called combination drugs. Combination drugs available in the United States as of early 2003 included Glucovance (glyburide and metformin), Avandamet (rosiglitazone and metformin), and Metaglip (glipizide and metformin).

Metformin is the common ingredient in all these drugs because it safely suppresses glucose production in the liver without the risk of hypoglycemia. The same risks and contraindications that apply to these drugs separately are also applicable to their combination formulation. However, even if you are familiar with one component of a combination drug (i.e., metformin), you should always read the drug's directions for use thoroughly before taking it to be aware of any unknown side effects or warnings.

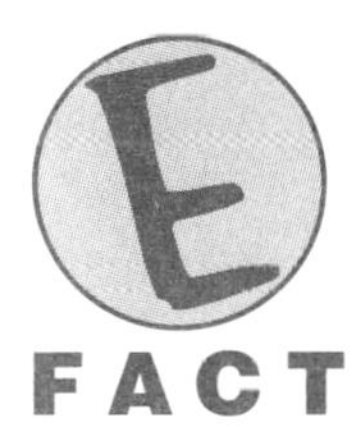

FACT

Several studies have shown that some diabetes drugs may have the potential to delay or prevent type 2 diabetes. Metformin reduced the risk of type 2 diabetes by 31 percent in the Diabetes Prevention Program (DPP), acarbose reduced the risk by 32 percent in the STOP-NIDDM trial, and troglitazone (now withdrawn from the market) reduced the risk by 56 percent in the TRIPOD study.

No Magic Pill

Prescription drugs are never a substitute for appropriate diet and exercise in the treatment of type 2 diabetes, and ignoring these other two fundamentals of diabetes management is a recipe for disaster. If and when you start medication, stay on track with your diet and exercise program. You need all three parts of the equation to manage your diabetes effectively.

On the other side of the coin, sometimes people with type 2 diabetes hesitate to agree to drugs because they feel like they have failed if they can't achieve blood glucose control with diet and exercise alone. Remember that medication is not a crutch, but just another tool for getting your blood glucose levels under control—your main objective in managing your diabetes. You need to take advantage of every tool at your disposal to build a solid and effective treatment program.

Chapter 10

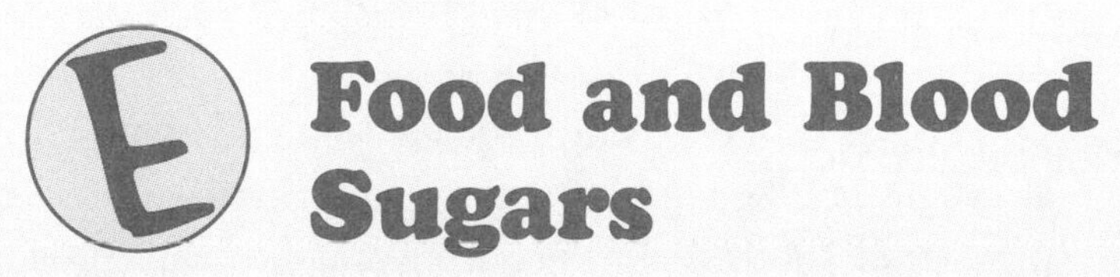

Food and Blood Sugars

Whether you're type 1 or type 2, the food you eat is going to have a major impact on your blood glucose levels and therefore on your diabetes control and risk of related complications. In fact, what you eat is so important that the ADA refers to dietary management of diabetes as "medical nutrition therapy" (MNT).

All about Carbohydrates

The body begins to convert carbohydrates almost entirely into glucose shortly after carb-containing foods are eaten. If you have inadequate or insufficient insulin to help process this glucose into cellular fuel, consuming too many carbohydrates can cause blood glucose to rise to dangerous levels. Without carbohydrate-generated glucose you could not function, yet too much can cause irreparable damage.

All foods that contain starches and/or sugars–including fruits, vegetables, milk, yogurt, breads, grains, beans, and pasta–contain carbs. Virtually the only whole foods that are carbohydrate-free are protein-rich meats, poultry, and finfish (when prepared without additional ingredients such as breading, marinade, or pickling) and fats such as cooking oils and shortening.

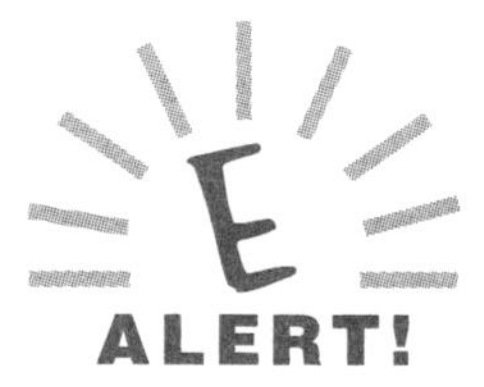

People with gastroparesis, or nerve damage of the stomach, have delayed stomach-emptying issues that causes the normal process of carbohydrate conversion to work differently. If you have gastroparesis or other gastrointestinal/digestive issues, make sure your dietitian is aware of them when working out a meal plan.

To avoid all carbohydrate-containing foods is both impossible and unadvisable–your body needs the important micronutrients and phytochemicals contained in these foods. In fact, the World Health Organization (WHO) recommends that carbohydrates from a variety of foods account for 55 percent of the total calories in your daily diet. But what you do need to learn is the basics of assessing the quantity and quality of carbohydrates in your food, and how your body reacts to them.

Carb Science

Carbohydrates are categorized by their chemical structure. A monosaccharide, or simple sugar, is composed of a single saccharide (sugar) chain. Glucose, fructose (fruit sugar), and galactose are all simple sugars. Disaccharides are two simple sugars joined together, and include lactose (milk sugar), maltose (malt sugar), and sucrose (table sugar). Polysaccharides, or complex carbohydrates, are ten or more simple sugar chains joined together. Glycogen, starches, and fiber are polysaccharides. (A fourth type of carbohydrate, oligosaccharides, is composed of three to ten sugar chains, but most of these are usually formed from the breakdown of polysaccharides.)

All carbohydrates are hydrolyzed, or broken down, into monosaccharides before they can be processed by the body. Amylase, a type of enzyme found in the saliva and secreted by the pancreas, helps to break down carbs into glucose during their journey through the small intestine. Once hydrolysis occurs, the resulting glucose is absorbed into the bloodstream. Any excess is converted to glycogen and stored in the liver.

The Glycemic Index

Does it matter what kind of carbs you consume? At one time, nutritionists believed that people with diabetes should avoid simple sugars (monosaccharides and disaccharides) and eat foods containing complex carbohydrates instead, with the mistaken belief that simple sugars would raise glucose levels faster and more dramatically across the board. But it's now known that gram for gram, complex carbohydrates found in breads, cereals, potatoes, vegetables, and other foods raise the blood sugar approximately the same amount as simple sugars like honey, fructose, or table sugar.

However, there may be a difference in how rapidly certain foods raise blood sugar levels. The glycemic index, or GI, is a measure of how quickly the carbs in certain foods are transformed into blood glucose. Foods with a low GI (e.g., beans, multigrain bread) raise glucose levels at a slower and steadier rate than a high-GI food (e.g., rice, potatoes).

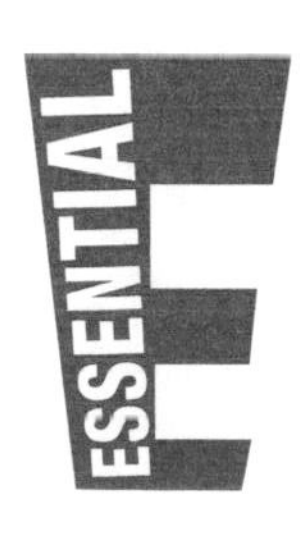

The GI of foods does not necessarily correspond to a specific carbohydrate "type"—some complex carbs may have a higher GI than simple carbs. For people with diabetes, the GI can be an effective tool for avoiding blood sugar spikes.

Carbs and Blood Glucose Control

Carbohydrates and the glucose they generate are an energy source—the dietary fuel of the human body. Insulin produced by the pancreas enables our cells to burn this carb-generated glucose. This is why determining the amount of carbohydrates in a meal is so important for blood sugar control.

People with type 1 diabetes, and some with type 2 diabetes, have to inject enough insulin to accommodate, or "cover," all the carbohydrates they eat. And many people with type 2 diabetes have the added task of having to adjust their diets to lose excess weight, as well. Concepts like carbohydrate counting and dietary exchanges, covered in the next chapter, enable people with diabetes to effectively manage their blood sugar levels.

It's also important to understand that carbohydrates don't work in isolation. Other nutrient components of the food you eat also can impact carb absorption. High-fat and high-protein foods can delay carb absorption. And although fiber is considered a carbohydrate, high-fiber foods also slow the absorption of glucose since they slow the passage of food through the digestive tract.

Why Fiber Is Important

Fiber, or roughage, is composed from plants' cell wall material. Whole grains, legumes (dried beans and peas), citrus fruits, nuts, and vegetables are all good sources of dietary fiber.

Fiber is considered a carbohydrate, but because it passes through the gastrointestinal system largely undigested, it does not effectively contribute to a rise in blood glucose levels. In fact, dietary fiber is an important nutritional tool in normalizing blood glucose levels because it slows digestion and therefore the absorption of accompanying nutrients.

How It Works

When viscous (water soluble) fiber absorbs water in the gastrointestinal tract, it turns to a gel-like, viscous substance that helps to normalize blood glucose and insulin levels by slowing the passage of food through the intestines. The delay in nutrient absorption means a slower and more stable rise in blood glucose levels.

Because it absorbs the excess intestinal bile acids that help to form cholesterol, soluble fiber has also been shown to help lower blood cholesterol levels, another important consideration in people with diabetes who are at risk for cardiovascular disease.

Another benefit is that viscous fiber improves satiety, or the feeling of fullness you get when eating a fiber-rich meal. It delays stomach emptying, and in those people with type 2 diabetes who are also overweight, satiety can be a useful tool for weight loss.

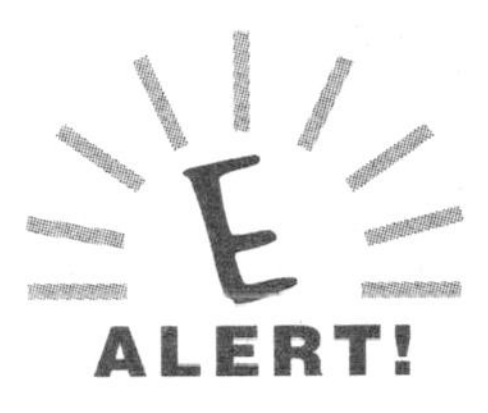

Always consume plenty of water or noncaffeinated beverages—at least 2 liters, or around eight glasses, daily—if you are eating a fiber-rich diet. Fiber without adequate fluids can lead to constipation. Increasing fiber intake slowly can also help to ease any bloating or other unwanted gastrointestinal distress.

Recommended Intake

A diet high in low-glycemic whole-grain cereal fiber has been found to have a beneficial effect in controlling postprandial (after meal) blood glucose levels and reducing serum cholesterol levels in people with type 2 diabetes. The ADA recommends a daily dietary intake of 20 to 35 grams of fiber, the same recommended dietary allowances (RDA) as for people without diabetes, to promote good control and cardiovascular health. However, some studies have shown a glucose- and lipid-lowering benefit with fiber intake of up to 50 grams daily. Talk to your doctor and dietitian about what level of fiber in your diet is right for you.

Fiber intake has also been associated with a reduction in diabetes risk in a number of studies. One of these, the six-year Nurses' Health Study, involving more than 65,000 participants, found that women on a low-fiber diet heavy in processed, sugary foods were 2.5 times more likely to develop type 2 diabetes than those who ate at least 25 grams of fiber daily.

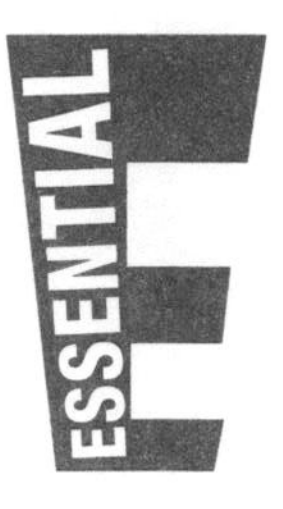

In the United States, carbohydrate information on food labels includes total dietary fiber (even though fiber is not digested). When counting carbs for the nutritional management of diabetes, total grams of dietary fiber should be subtracted from total carbohydrates.

Sugar Is Not the Enemy

The no-sugar myth is probably one of the biggest misconceptions about diabetes. The reality is that it isn't sugar specifically that raises blood glucose levels—it's any food containing carbohydrates, including honey, fruit, milk, and vegetables, to name a few. So whether it's a spoonful of sugar, a bagel, or a banana, it will cause blood sugar levels to rise. The reason some people with diabetes prefer to use sugar substitutes such as artificial sweeteners or sugar alcohols is because they contain little to no carbohydrates or calories.

Sugar Alcohols

A sugar alcohol is, quite simply, a monosaccharide that has been chemically transformed into its alcohol form. There are a number of naturally occurring sugar alcohols (also called polyols), including sorbitol, mannitol, xylitol, lactitol, maltitol, isomalt, erythritol, and hydrogenated starch hydrolysates. Because they are not completely absorbed in the gastrointestinal tract, the rise in blood glucose levels that they cause is less than with sucrose, which is why people with diabetes may find them desirable. Polyols are frequently used as a sweetener and bulking agent in processed foods marketed as sugar-free.

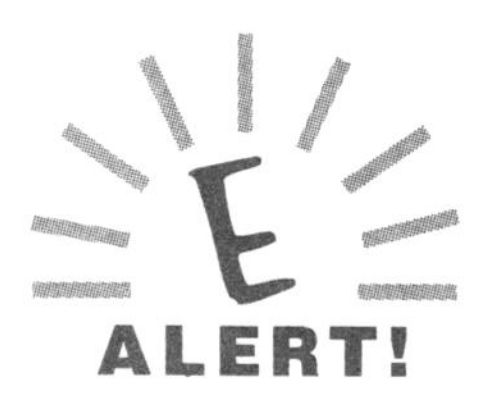

Because children have a lower tolerance for sugar alcohol sweeteners, check the labels of "sugar-free" foods carefully and be cautious with the amount of sugar alcohols your child consumes.

Some people find that sugar alcohols have a laxative effect, causing diarrhea and/or gas. The U.S. Food and Drug Administration requires that foods containing significant amounts of sorbitol or mannitol (those products where daily consumption may result in over 50 grams of sorbitol or 20 grams of mannitol) must be labeled with the statement: "Excess consumption may have a laxative effect."

Artificial Sweeteners

As opposed to naturally derived sugar alcohols, artificial sweeteners are synthetically manufactured sugar substitutes:

- **Aspartame (NutraSweet or Equal):** This FDA-approved sweetener is 180 times sweeter than table sugar. Aspartame has been the subject of much controversy regarding potential health effects, but there is currently ***no*** clinical research that indicates that the sweetener is unsafe for most people (except for individuals with advanced liver disease, pregnant women with hyperphenylalanine, or high levels of phenylalanine in the bloodstream, and those with a rare genetic condition known as *phenylketonuria*, or PKU).
- **Neotame:** This sweetener is derived from aspartic acid and phenylalanine (both are amino acids). Neotame is considered safe for use in people with diabetes, children, pregnant and lactating women, and individuals with PKU.
- **Saccharin (Sweet 'n Low):** The oldest artificial sweetener, saccharin was discovered in 1879 and has been used as a sweetener in foods and beverages for over a century. Saccharin has been linked to bladder cancer in rats, but there is no hard data establishing that normal amounts of the sweetener are dangerous for humans. In 2000, based on a newer and more relevant body of human studies, the National Toxicology Program of the National Institutes of Health took saccharin off their ninth edition of the Report of Carcinogens list and President Clinton signed legislation removing the carcinogenic warning label from saccharin-containing products. Saccharin is considered GRAS (or generally recognized as safe) by the FDA, and is about 300 times sweeter than table sugar.

- **Acesulfame potassium (Sunett):** Acesulfame potassium, also called acesulfame K, is FDA approved for use as a sweetener in processed foods and beverages. It is an estimated 200 times sweeter than table sugar, and studies have confirmed its safe use in people with diabetes, pregnant and nursing women, children, and the general population.
- **Sucralose (Splenda):** Sucralose is unique in that it is actually derived from table sugar. However, unlike table sugar it has no carbohydrates, no calories, and it passes through the body almost entirely undigested. The sugar substitute, which is 600 times sweeter than table sugar, was cleared by the FDA for use as a food additive and a sweetener in the late 1990s. Because it is very stable and withstands temperature changes well, it can be used in cooking and baking. Extensive clinical studies have uncovered no safety risks for people with diabetes and the general population.

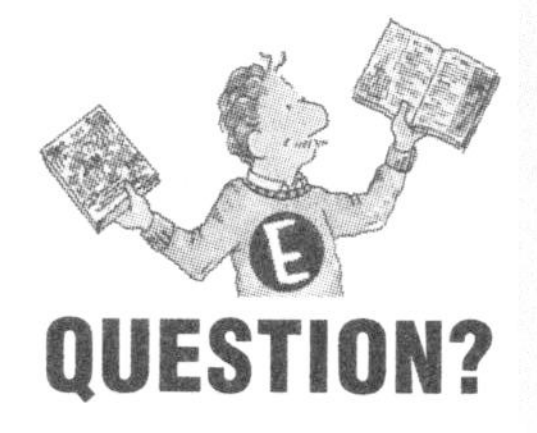

QUESTION?

If it's sugar-free, does that mean I can eat as much as I want?
Don't be misled by a "sugar-free" label. Foods containing polyols and/or artificial sweeteners may still contain carbohydrates and calories that should be figured into your meal plan. Read the nutrition facts on the label to get the full story.

A Few Words on Stevia

Stevia is a dietary supplement derived from the herb *Stevia rebaudiana*, a wild shrub that is grown in South America and the Pacific Rim. Although used extensively as a sweetener for food products throughout South America and Asia, stevia is not approved for use in the United States, Canada, or the European Union. The FDA initially banned the import of the herb in 1991, following a study that raised questions about its toxicity as a food additive, but subsequently allowed it to be sold as a dietary supplement. However, the FDA has refused to add it to its GRAS list, citing a lack of substantial, controlled data on the safety of the herb.

Because stevia does not affect blood glucose levels, it is often touted as a sweetener alternative for people with diabetes. The extract of the herb (called steviosides) is said to be 200 to 300 times sweeter than table sugar and is used in cooking and baking outside the United States. Extracts are available in powder, tablet, liquid, and capsule form. Stevia is also available in a green herbal powder formula that is less intense than the extract. Both types of stevia are available in health food stores, again marketed as dietary supplements.

If you're considering using stevia, talk with your doctor and dietitian before incorporating it into your food plan. A dietitian familiar with the herb can also provide information on sugar to stevia conversion for cooking.

Caloric Intake

Ideal calorie intake is based on your activity level, gender, age, and other factors. Many people with type 2 diabetes also face weight-loss challenges; since reducing calorie intake is one component of an effective weight-reduction program, it is an important consideration in dietary management of diabetes.

The following are the average daily calorie RDAs for different genders, age groups, and activity levels (derived from USDA data):

- Children 2 to 6—1,600 calories daily
- Children 7 to 12—2,200 calories daily
- Teen girls—2,200 calories daily
- Teen boys—2,800 calories daily
- Active women—2,200 calories daily
- Sedentary women—1,600 calories daily
- Active men—2,800 calories daily
- Sedentary men—2,200 calories daily
- Women over 50—1,900 calories daily
- Men over 50—2,500 calories daily

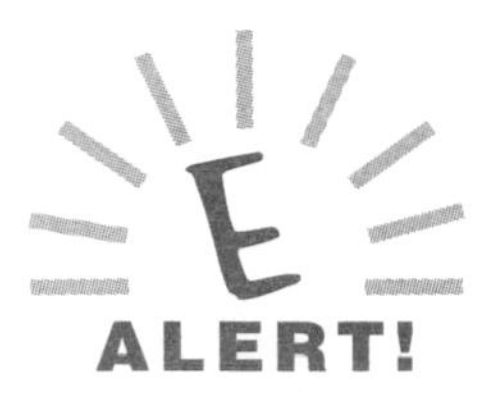

Keep in mind that these are just general guidelines. For example, athletes who expend more energy may require more calories, and children who are inactive due to a health condition will probably require less. You should speak with your dietitian about calorie requirements that are right for you.

It's More Than Just the Calories

If you are overweight and have type 2 diabetes, keep in mind that even modest weight loss can decrease insulin resistance and improve control. But calorie reduction alone rarely leads to long-term weight control. The ADA recommends a comprehensive approach of reduced calories (500 to 1,000 fewer than the RDA for weight maintenance), regular exercise, reduced fat intake (no more than 30 percent of daily calories from fat), and diabetes and weight management education for long-term success. Chapter 13 covers diabetes and weight loss in greater detail.

The nutrient balance in the food your calories come from is also important. No more than 30 percent of total calories should come from fat. The ADA suggests that carbohydrates and monounsaturated fat together should account for 60 to 70 percent of total calories.

Fats and Cholesterol

Fat insulates the body and supplies energy when no carbohydrate sources are available. It also enables the body to absorb and process the fat-soluble vitamins A, D, E, and K. However, too much saturated fat and cholesterol can increase the risk of atherosclerosis and other cardiovascular complications from diabetes.

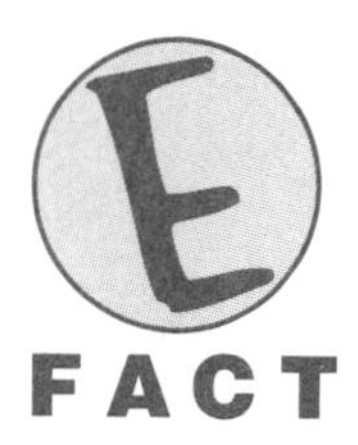
FACT

The dietary supplement chromium picolinate has demonstrated an insulin-enhancing effect in several clinical studies, though most available information suggests that it does not help in reducing elevated glucose levels in type 2 diabetes. Before taking any supplement, always consult your physician.

All Fats Are Not Created Equal

Fats are confusing to many people when they first start learning the ropes about dietary management of diabetes. The off-target message that all fat is bad has entrenched itself in popular dietary culture; fat-free food production is now a multimillion-dollar industry. While some fats are bad for you in excess, others can actually help improve your cholesterol profile. Here are the basics on dietary fats:

- **Saturated fat:** Solid fats that are found in meat and dairy products and vegetable oils. They are associated with high LDL (bad) cholesterol levels.
- **Unsaturated fat:** Either polyunsaturated (e.g., safflower oil) or monounsaturated (e.g., olive oil). Fish and seafood are good sources of unsaturated fat. These types of fats (polyunsaturated in particular) have been shown to be effective in reducing total and LDL (bad) cholesterol levels.
- **Transfats/hydrogenated fats:** Transunsaturated fatty acids, or unsaturated liquid fats that have been processed into a more saturated and solid form by adding hydrogen. They are often found in processed baked goods and commercial fried foods, and may be called "partially hydrogenated" or "hydrogenated" fats. Transfatty acids can raise LDL (bad) cholesterol and lower HDL (good) cholesterol, and their use should be limited.
- **Essential fatty acids:** Fish and fish oils and certain seeds and nuts and their oils (e.g., flaxseed, canola, soybean, and walnut) are all good sources of omega-3 fatty acids, which have heart-protective benefits and lower both triglyceride levels and blood pressure. Linolenic, alpha-linolenic, eicosapentaenoic, and docosahexaenoic acids are all essential fatty acids.
- **Dietary cholesterol:** Cholesterol is present in food that comes from animals, including poultry, fish, eggs, meats, and dairy products.

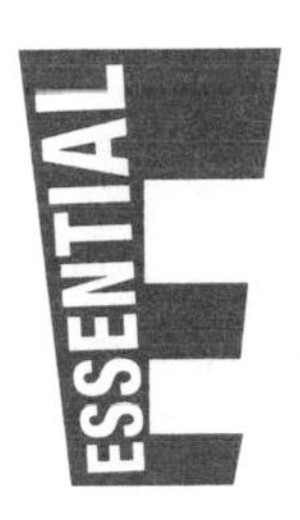

Although monounsaturated and especially polyunsaturated fats can be helpful in lowering LDL and triglyceride levels, they should still be eaten in moderation. Fats have twice the calories of protein and carbohydrates (9 calories per gram versus approximately 4), and too much of any kind will widen your waistline, guaranteed.

Less than 10 percent of daily calories should come from saturated fats. The ADA suggests that people with LDL cholesterol of 100 mg/dl or higher may benefit from lowering saturated fat intake even lower (to less than 7 percent of calories). They also recommend two to three servings of fish weekly for the cardioprotective benefits of omega-3 fatty acids. Daily cholesterol intake should be 300 milligrams or less (and less than 200 milligrams per day for those with an LDL cholesterol level of 100 mg/dl or higher).

Fake Fats

Fat substitutes are food additives derived from protein, carbohydrates, or chemically modified fat. They are designed to replace the texture, moisture-retention, and bulk of fat in food while contributing a lower amount of calories. The main pitfall of reduced-fat and fat-free foods is that some people interpret the label as meaning calorie-free and overindulge. However, when prudently used, reduced-fat products can be a useful component of a weight-loss plan. Both the ADA and the American Heart Association (AHA) agree that further studies are needed to determine the long-term impact of fat substitutes on overall calorie intake and nutrient absorption.

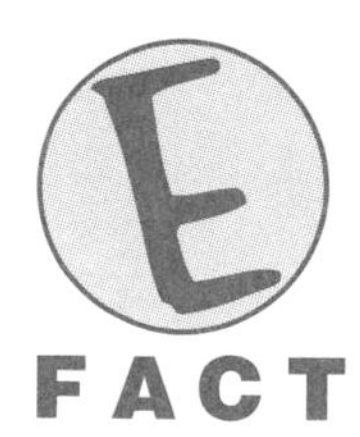

FACT

Food with high fat and/or high protein levels can delay the absorption of carbohydrates, and consequently the postprandial (after meal) rise of blood glucose. People who take insulin need to be especially aware of this phenomenon, as taking insulin too early can result in unwanted highs or lows. Pizza is one food that is well known for causing this "delayed reaction" in people with diabetes.

Some fat substitutes, such as olestra (Olean), may inhibit the absorption of fat-soluble vitamins A, D, E, and K. The FDA has mandated that products made with olestra be fortified with these vitamins to overcome the deficit.

Protein and Diabetes

Proteins are chains of amino acids responsible for cell growth and maintenance and are found in virtually every part of the body. Protein in foods from animal sources (meat, poultry, fish, and dairy) is called complete protein because it contains essential amino acids necessary for building and maintaining cells. Plant-based foods such as grains, beans, fruit, and vegetables contain incomplete proteins, with only partial groups of these amino acids. However, different incomplete plant-based proteins can be combined to form complete proteins in the diet. If you are a vegetarian or vegan and have diabetes, a dietitian with experience in vegetarian menu planning can advise you on appropriate protein consumption.

People with diabetes should have the same 10 to 15 percent of total calories from protein that are recommended for the general population. The exception to this is people with impaired kidney function, or nephropathy. Because damaged kidneys cannot filter protein efficiently from the bloodstream, these individuals may benefit from a low-protein diet. If you have kidney problems, talk to your doctor and dietitian about an appropriate level of protein for your diet.

Sensible Sodium Intake

In moderate amounts, dietary sodium or sodium chloride (salt) is not harmful. In fact, the mineral helps to maintain a healthy electrolyte balance and works in tandem with potassium to regulate blood acid/base balance, heart function, nerve impulses, and muscle contractions.

However, people with high blood pressure need to be cautious about having too much sodium in their daily diet. Sodium acts as a vasoconstrictor, constricting (or tightening) blood vessels, which can elevate blood pressure even further. For people with diabetes and hypertension, the ADA recommends a reduction in sodium intake to 2,400 milligrams (100 mmol). That recommendation is equivalent to 6,000 milligrams (6 grams, or just over a teaspoon) of sodium chloride. The average American, however, consumes over twice that much.

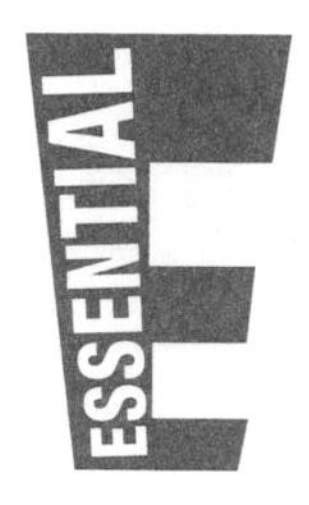

When calculating your sodium intake, be sure to include the sodium in processed foods as well as the salt you add to your food. Be on the lookout for monosodium glutamate (MSG), sodium nitrite (nitrate), sodium caseinate, sodium alginate, sodium sulfite, sodium hydroxinate, sodium propionate, sodium saccharin, sodium bicarbonate (baking soda), and sodium benzoate. Even some multivitamins contain sodium.

Some people with diabetes and hypertension may benefit from an even bigger cut in dietary salt. A 2001 study published in the *New England Journal of Medicine* examined sodium intake in the Dietary Approaches to Stop Hypertension (DASH) diet and found that reducing sodium intake to levels below the current recommendation of 2,400 milligrams per day to 1,560 milligrams (65 mmol) and 960 milligrams (40 mmol) reduces blood pressure significantly when it is part of a comprehensive DASH diet—a dietary approach low in saturated fat and cholesterol and rich in fiber, protein, calcium, magnesium, and potassium. Ⓔ

Chapter 11

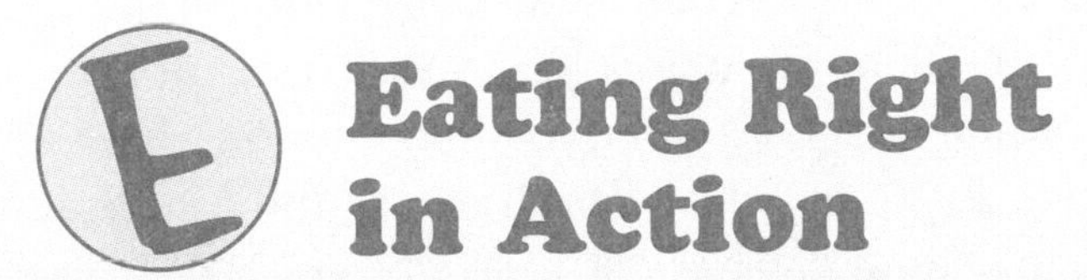

Eating Right in Action

If you're looking for a "diabetic diet" full of bland, boring foods and completely devoid of any desserts, indulgences, or the other little taste treats that make life worth living, you are out of luck. The so-called diabetic diet is largely a myth; people with diabetes can and do enjoy a wide variety of foods, the same foods everyone else can eat. The key is moderation, a focus on healthier food choices, and a keener awareness of how foods affect your blood sugars and body.

Menu Planning

A meeting with a registered dietitian is an absolute must for anyone with diabetes. A good RD will explain the mysteries of exchanges and carbohydrate counting to you and will work with you to create a meal plan that works with your lifestyle. Parents cooking for a child with type 1 diabetes will have a whole different set of concerns and dietary issues than, for example, an adult with type 2 who wants to learn how to eat for better control when he's out on the road. If you don't have an RD already, talk to your doctor about a referral, or visit the American Dietetic Association's online referral database at *www.eatright.org*.

As part of your diabetes care team, your dietitian should be in close contact with your care provider. Make sure she's on top of any adjustments to your insulin or medication, which go hand in hand with what you're eating. The dietitian's office is another of those places where it helps to bring a spouse or companion for another set of ears, particularly your first time there.

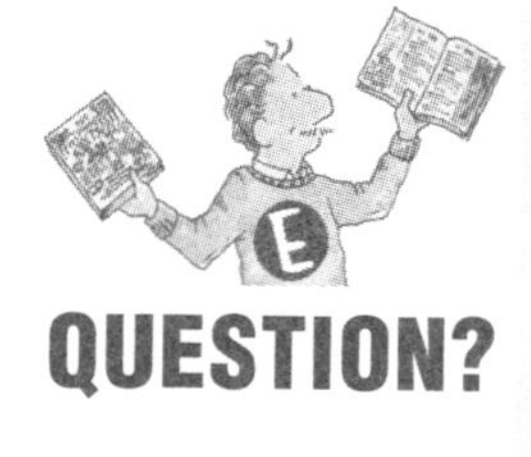

QUESTION?

I'm trying hard to manage my type 2 diabetes through diet and exercise, but my wife continues to buy my favorite junk food for the kids. How can I eat right with that around?
Diabetes is a family disease. Ask your wife to join you for a diabetes education class and/or a meeting with your dietitian and discuss ways of promoting a healthier lifestyle for the entire family. Your children will actually benefit from the same type of healthy meal plan you're following for your diabetes.

Whether you're using exchanges or carbohydrate counting, your RD will try to spread out your carbohydrate intake more or less evenly throughout the day to promote blood glucose balance. Again, your dietitian will work with you to come up with an appropriate amount of exchanges or carb grams, fat intake, and protein. He may also suggest other dietary guidelines based on your health history (e.g., low sodium if you have hypertension).

On average, you will probably be eating between 40 to 55 percent of your total daily calories in the form of carbohydrates. A 1,600-calorie diet that is 50 percent carbs, for example, would contain 800 calories from carbs. That translates to 200 grams of carbs (1 gram carb equals 4 calories), or just about thirteen carb exchanges/choices for the day. Remember that this is an average. Some people with diabetes may find that a lower percentage of carbs offers them better control.

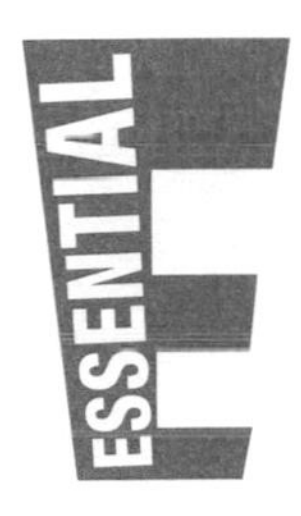

Low-carb, high-protein diets have soared in popularity thanks to medical media icons like the late Dr. Atkins. However, the jury is still out on their long-term safety. People with kidney impairment should avoid any diet that is heavy on protein, as it can worsen the condition. If you'd like to try a lower-carb meal plan, talk with your RD and your doctor about a safe approach that's right for you.

Diabetes Food Pyramid

It's important to include a variety of vegetables, fruits, grains, and other nutrient-dense foods in your diet. The ADA suggests a slightly modified version of the USDA food pyramid as a guideline for daily servings. The only difference is that starchy vegetables are moved out of the vegetable portion and down into the breads at the base of the pyramid with the rest of the starch-heavy foods. The general daily guidelines are as follows:

- Breads, grains, legumes, and starchy vegetables: 6 to 11 servings
- Nonstarchy vegetables: 3 to 5 servings
- Fruits: 2 to 4 servings
- Milk and yogurt: 2 to 3 servings
- Meat and meat substitutes (proteins): 2 to 3 servings
- Fats and sweets: Use sparingly

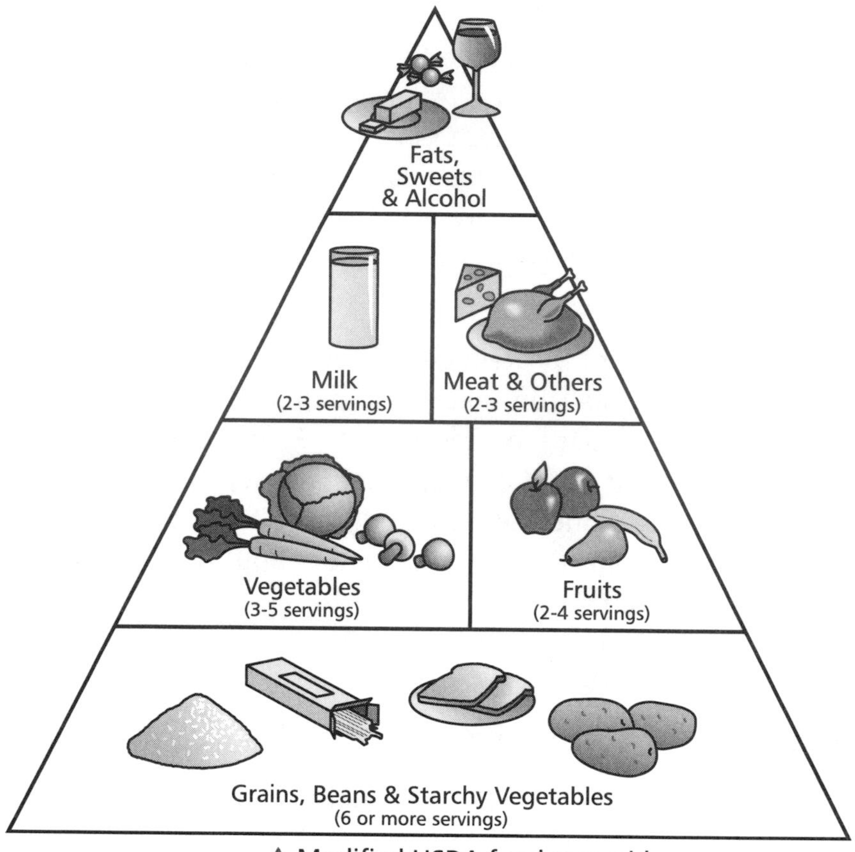

▲ Modified USDA food pyramid

The Harvard School of Public Health has a different opinion on what you should be eating, using carbohydrate quality as a blueprint. The Healthy Eating Food Pyramid pushes starchy, high-glycemic index carbs up to the top of the pyramid and adds heart-healthy oils to the whole grains at the bottom:

- Unprocessed whole grains and healthy oils (e.g., canola, olive, safflower): 6 to 11 servings
- Nonstarchy vegetables: In abundance
- Fruits: 3 to 5 servings
- Nuts and legumes: 1 to 2 servings
- Dairy: 1 to 2 servings
- Fish, poultry, and eggs: 0 to 2 servings
- Refined grains, high-carb starches, butter, red meat, and sweets: Use sparingly

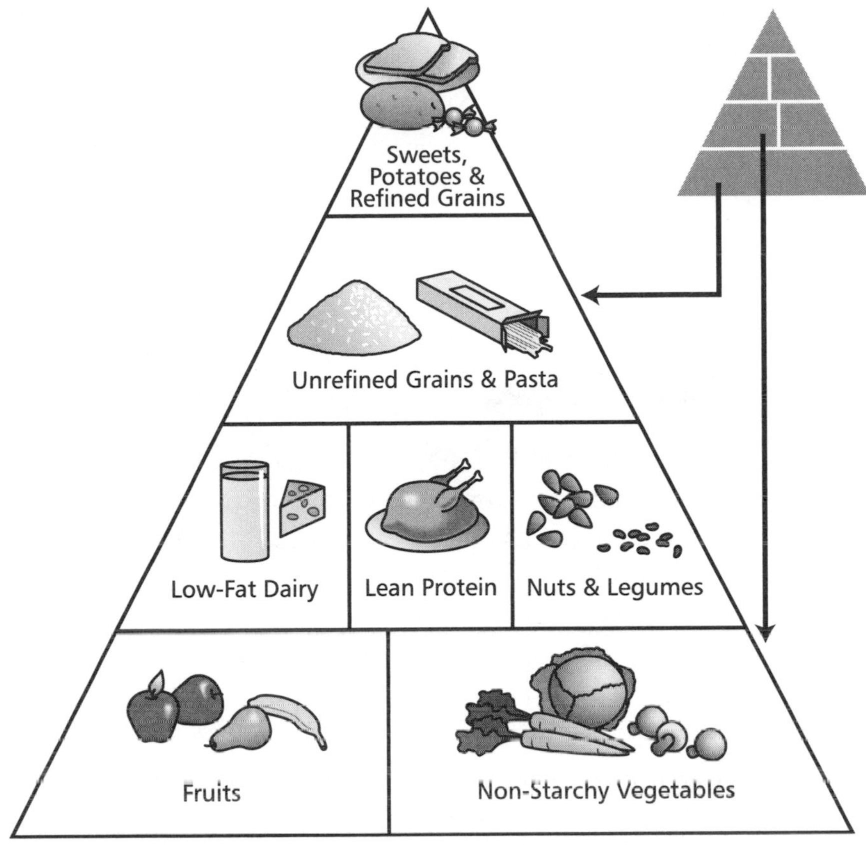

▲ Healthy eating food pyramid

Adapted from "A Low Glycemic Index Pyramid" by David S. Ludwig, MD, Ph.D., Children's Hospital, Boston.

Dear Diary . . .

Even if you follow your meal plan to the letter, you're still going to find that certain foods will give you a bigger spike in glucose levels than expected. You may also find that other foods you expected to pump up your readings barely bump the meter. That's the individual nature of diabetes. For this reason, a food diary is an invaluable tool in figuring out just how different foods affect your blood glucose levels.

Record the type, amount, and timing of foods eaten, along with what affect they had on your blood glucose levels (a reading before eating and a reading two-hours postprandial). Many people choose to record the information in their blood glucose logbook. At first it may feel a little obsessive-compulsive to chronicle every bite, but you'll find it's worth it when the time comes to figure out a mysterious high or an unexpected low. It's also a great cure for mindless eating—you won't be polishing off what the kids left on their dinner plate or munching samples in the supermarket if you've trained yourself to write it down.

Dietary Exchanges

One time-tested method of managing your diabetes through diet is the dietary exchange system. The exchange lists are a team effort by the American Diabetes Association and the American Dietetic Association (the two ADAs). There are three food group types represented in the exchange lists—the carbohydrate group, the meat and meat substitutes group, and the fat group. Each list within each group contains foods with a similar carbohydrate, protein, fat, and calorie content.

Dietary Exchanges

	Carbohydrates	Protein	Fat	Calories
	Carbohydrate Group			
Starch	15 g	3 g	0–1 g	80
Fruit	15 g	–	–	60
Nonstarchy veggies	5 g	2 g	–	25
Milk, fat-free/low-fat	12 g	8 g	0–3 g	90
Milk, reduced-fat	12 g	8 g	5 g	120
Milk, whole	12 g	8 g	8 g	150
Other carbs (sweets, etc.)	15 g	varies	varies	varies

Dietary Exchanges				
	Carbohydrates	Protein	Fat	Calories
Meat and Meat Substitutes Group				
Very lean	–	7 g	0–1 g	35
Lean	–	7 g	3 g	55
Medium-fat	–	7 g	5 g	75
High-fat	–	7 g	8 g	100
Fat Group (Oils, Nuts, Etc.)				
All fats	–	–	5 g	45

The exchange system also has a category called the free foods group. Free foods are those that contain 5 grams or fewer of carbohydrates and/or have fewer than 20 calories.

When you sit down with your dietitian, she will work with you to specify a certain number of each type of exchanges for your meals based on your caloric requirements and nutritional needs. You can think of exchanges like trading cards. Any food on a particular list can be swapped with another on the same list. So if you have one fruit exchange allotted for a snack and have a taste for fresh fruit instead of the juice you had planned, you could trade your ½ cup of orange juice for 1 cup of raspberries, as both have a roughly equivalent carb, fat, and protein value. Remember that you only trade within lists, not across lists. You can't trade a fruit exchange for a fat exchange, for example.

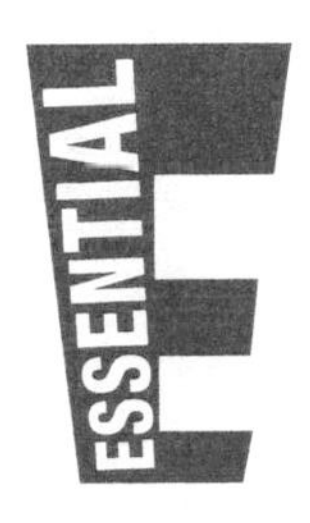

The exchange lists are based on averages. For whole foods like fruit and vegetables, you'll find them fairly accurate. Because of variances in food processing and ingredients, you should check the nutritional values of anything you buy with a label to ensure that they are still roughly equivalent to the exchanges you use.

Some people say they find the exchange system limiting because of the finite number of foods on the "official" exchange lists. Take a walk on the wild side and try something exotic. As long as you have the nutritional breakdown of the food, either on the label or through a food guide or database, you can compute the exchanges. There are software programs and nutritional calculators that can do the math for you. You can also purchase the official exchange lists from either ADA organization for a nominal fee.

For those who like to cook, exchanges can also be computed for mixed meals like casseroles, stews, and soups by totaling the carb, protein, fat, and calories for each ingredient and dividing by the number of servings—the result may be translated into exchanges. You will have to use your measuring tools, however; if you are the "pinch of this, dash of that" type, try to reign in your compulsion and use that food scale. There are dozens of excellent diabetes cookbooks on the market that list full nutritional breakdowns with recipes; *The Everything® Diabetes Cookbook* by Pamela Rice Hahn (Adams Media, 2002) is a good choice.

Carbohydrate Counting

If you find exchange lists tedious or feel math-challenged, carbohydrate counting may be a good option for you. Carb counting involves calculating the grams of carbohydrate eaten in a given meal. In theory, regulating carb intake means controlling your blood glucose levels.

How many carbohydrates you eat in a given day depends on your unique caloric, medical, and lifestyle needs. An active teenager will have a greater carbohydrate requirement than an inactive adult. Again, the first step in establishing a carb-counting plan is sitting down with a registered dietitian who will discuss your medical history, lifestyle, eating habits, and medication routines, and come up with a plan for how many carbohydrates you should be eating and when they should be consumed.

Choices Versus Grams

There are a couple of different variations on the carb-counting theme. Basic carb gram counting is simply calculating the actual grams of carbohydrates consumed and ensuring they don't exceed a pre-established limit. Another popular method is carb choice.

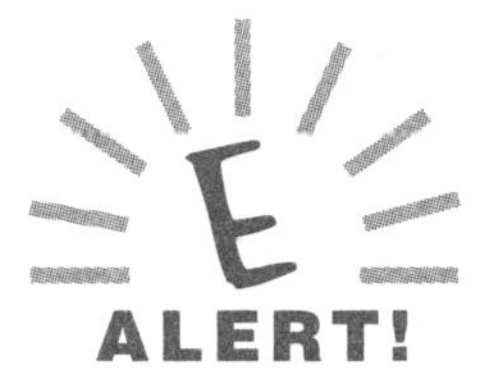

As you learn how variations in food choices, timing of meals, and exercise affect your blood glucose levels, you and your dietitian and doctor can work together to fine-tune your carb-counting program. It is a learning process, so don't be disappointed if it doesn't fall into place immediately for you.

Since a dietary exchange of starch or fruit carbohydrates is equivalent to 15 grams of carbohydrates, many dietitians use the "15 grams per serving" value as a "rule of thumb" in teaching carb counting, especially to those patients who are already familiar with exchange lists. Each 15-gram serving is called a "carb choice," and instead of establishing a total number of carbohydrate grams for the day, you will work with your dietitian to determine a total number of carb choices. The Carb Choices table shows how to translate exchanges into carb choices.

Carb Choices

Exchange Equivalent	Carb Grams	Carb Choices
1 starch	15 g	1 carb choice
1 fruit	12 g	1 carb choice
3 nonstarchy vegetables	15 g	1 carb choice
1 milk	12 g	1 carb choice
other carbs	15 g	1 carb choice
meat	0 g	0 carb choices
fat	0 g	0 carb choices

The choice method may not be as exact as calculating carbs strictly by the label, since it involves a certain degree of estimation, but it's close enough for most people. Talk to your dietitian about the method that works best for you.

Carb counting can also take some practice. In the United States, all food labeling must list carbohydrate content on a per serving basis, so the carb content in packaged foods is easy to determine. It's important to remember that FDA-prescribed serving sizes and the portions you are used to may often be two very different things. Make sure you account for any extra carbs in bigger servings.

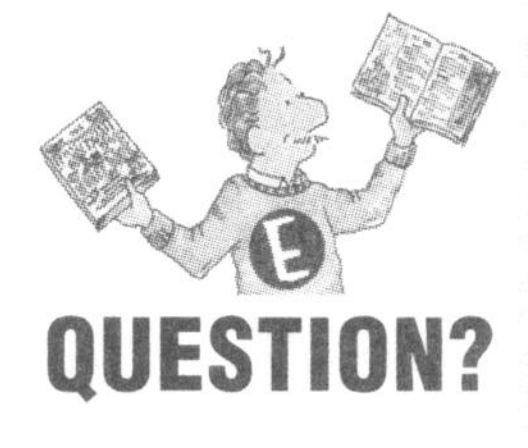

QUESTION?

My nutritionist told me that 15 grams of carbohydrate is equal to one serving, but that doesn't always match the serving size information on the food labels I read. Which is right?
Both, of course! For example, a half-cup of apple juice has 15 grams of carbohydrates and is equivalent to one carb choice serving, but the carbs for the 1-cup serving size indicated on the label would be twice that (30 grams, or two carb choice servings). Make sure you know how many carbs you are consuming in your serving size.

A good carbohydrate-counting reference book for fresh whole foods is also a must. Even if you don't cook from scratch, you'll need to know the carb counts in those fruits and veggies, and a carb guide may also be useful for when you're eating out and don't have the benefits of checking labels.

Advanced Carb Counting

Carbohydrate counting can offer people who use insulin more control and greater flexibility in what they eat. If you use a fast-acting insulin like Humalog or NovoLog prior to a meal, you can determine how many units you need to take based on both your blood glucose reading prior to the meal and on the number of carbohydrate grams you plan on eating. This is referred to as "covering" your carbohydrates.

The starting point for this insulin to carbohydrate ratio is about 1:15 (1 unit of insulin for every 15 grams of carbs on the menu). Along with covering the carbohydrates, an additional unit of insulin should be added for every 50 mg/dl that blood sugar is above the target range. For example, if you had 60 grams of carbs on your lunch menu, and your blood glucose levels were 100 mg/dl over your target goal prior to the meal, you would inject 6 units of insulin (4 for the carbs and 2 for the blood glucose). Your mileage may vary; by logging your glucose levels regularly and tracking reactions to meals and insulin, you and your provider should be able to fine-tune your specific ratios.

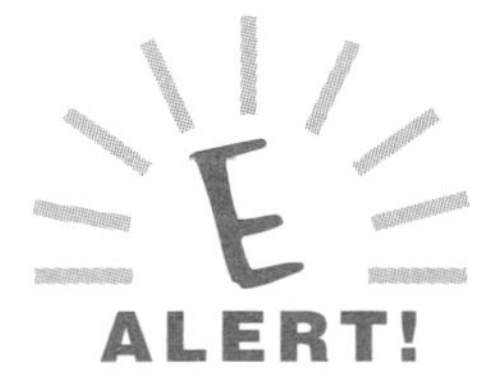

When you're planning on enjoying a high-fiber meal or snack, you must adjust your insulin dose accordingly. For any meal with more than 5 grams of fiber, you need to subtract the total fiber from the total carbs *before* computing your insulin dose.

People who are more insulin resistant may require a larger amount of insulin than those who still retain a great deal of insulin sensitivity. There are several methods for computing insulin sensitivity and insulin to carbohydrate ratio; for more information, see Chapter 8.

Glycemic Index (GI)

While carbohydrate counting is based on the idea that all carbs are created equal, and it is the total number of carb grams, not the type of carb (i.e., simple or complex; starch or fruit) that is the bottom line for blood sugar control, the glycemic index takes a different tack, looking at carb quality instead of quantity.

The GI is a measure of how quickly a carbohydrate affects blood glucose levels. High-GI foods cause quick spikes, while low-GI foods provide a slower, steadier release of glucose. In general, unprocessed, fiber-rich foods tend to be the lowest on the GI scale, while processed and starch-heavy carbohydrates are the highest.

To determine the glycemic index of a food, researchers give a test subject some quantity of the food that contains 50 grams of carbs, and then their blood glucose levels are measured at regular intervals to determine how quickly the carbs in the food turn into glucose. That response is then measured against a standard value of how quickly 50 grams of either glucose or white bread (both 100 on the GI scale) causes blood glucose to rise, and is expressed as a percentage between 1 and 140. The results among a group of testers (usually ten) are averaged to come up with the GI.

Using the GI

Some people with diabetes use the GI as a reference guide for choosing slow, low-GI carbs to keep glucose levels under control and avoid blood sugar spikes. High-GI foods also have their place. If you're about to go for a quick sprint, you'd want to make sure a pre-exercise carb snack provides the quick release of energy you need. And a fast-acting, high GI carb is preferable over a low one for treating a hypo.

One important caveat to using the GI as your guide—don't become so carb-centric that you lose sight of your overall nutrient intake. The lower-GI food may not always be the best choice; a Snickers bar has a GI of 44 while a bowl of Cheerios has a GI of 74. Although this may be your perfect justification for satisfying your sweet tooth, it's obvious that the healthier choice here is the cereal. Keep your vitamins, minerals, protein, and fat intake in perspective.

Glycemic Load

Another anomaly of the GI is that the system doesn't make adjustments for the quantity of carbs per serving. Some foods with a high index value simply don't contain enough carbohydrates per serving to make much of an impact on glucose levels. You'd have to eat over six servings of cooked beets to get the same amount of carbohydrates in one large baked potato, yet both have a relatively high GI (91 and 121, respectively).

Researchers at the Harvard School of Public Health have come up with a way to bridge this quality versus quantity gap—the *glycemic load.* To compute glycemic load of a food, convert its GI percentage value into decimal format (i.e., 91 is equivalent to .91) and multiply it by the grams of carbohydrates in one serving. At first glance, you might want to pass up beets based on their GI alone, despite the fact that they are an excellent source of folate and potassium. But although the GI of cooked beets is 91, a ½-cup serving only has 8.46 grams of carbs. That makes its glycemic load only 7.69 (.91 × 8.46). By comparison, a carb-dense large baked potato has 50.96 carbohydrates (with skin), a GI of 121, and a whopping glycemic load of 62.

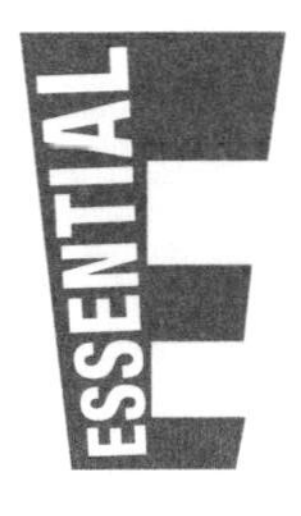

Food GI is not set in stone. Raw foods may have a different GI than the same food cooked; preparation methods can also impact GI. Fruits may have a lower or higher GI depending on their stage of ripeness. Some foods will not have a GI, and it isn't unusual for the GI of processed foods to vary by brand. In addition, one version of GI uses white bread for the reference food, while the other uses glucose.

It's Not Easy

GI is a good tool for making smart food choices. However, it does require a motivated patient who isn't scared of a little math. And because GI is not something listed on food labels, it requires a small investment in a book of GI listings. Dr. Jennie Brand-Miller and Dr. Thomas Wolever are considered two of the world's leading authorities on the GI, and have authored what is arguably the best of the bunch—*The New Glucose Revolution* (Marlowe & Co., 2002). There are also several lists and GI databases available online (see Appendix A for more information).

In part because of its relative complexity, the American Diabetes Association has not endorsed the use of the glycemic index as a strategy for meal planning. The ADA also cites the lack of controlled studies showing the benefits of a low-GI diet in lowering long-term HbA1c, although they do acknowledge that using the GI can result in lower postprandial blood glucose readings. However, both the World Health Organization and the European Association for the Study of Diabetes recommend its use for the nutritional management of diabetes. If you're interested in trying the GI yourself, talk with your dietitian or doctor about how to incorporate it into your meal plan.

Weights and Measures: Portion Control

You can't measure every morsel that passes your lips, but it's a good idea to measure most foods and beverages until you get a feel for portion sizes. It's a supersized world out there, and most people are surprised to find that their idea of a single serving is actually two or three.

If you're into bells and whistles, there are food scales that are preprogrammed with nutritional information, as well as scales that will keep a running total of your daily food and nutrient intake for you. The only tools you really need, however, are a simple and inexpensive gram scale, dry and liquid measuring cups, and measuring spoons. Early on, it's a good idea to run everything that isn't premeasured through a scale, cup, or spoon first.

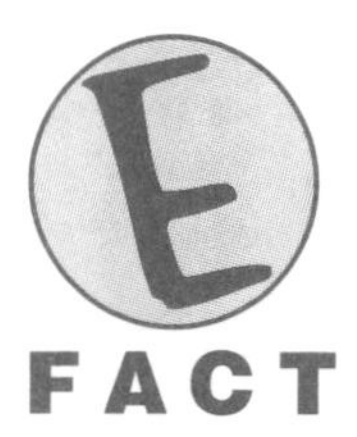

FACT

Americans are eating substantially more. A 2003 study published in the *Journal of the American Medical Association* found that portion sizes of the "all-American foods" studied—salty snacks, desserts, soft drinks, fruit drinks, French fries, hamburgers, cheeseburgers, pizza, and Mexican food—grew considerably for all foods except pizza, most notably at fast-food restaurants and at the dinner table.

Ballparking It

Get intimate with your food, or rather, your dishes. Have a favorite mug or bowl? Pay attention to how completely a serving of yogurt or soup fills it up. You'll soon that find it's second nature to guesstimate your portion sizes.

There will be times when you can't use your favorite cup. Pulling out a gram scale at your favorite restaurant is a little unrealistic. In these cases, it helps to have some rough equivalents for comparison.

Here are some typical serving sizes and some points of reference for estimating portion sizes:

- A cup of fruit or yogurt–a baseball, a clenched fist, or a small apple
- Three ounces of fish, meat, or poultry–a deck of cards, the palm of your hand, or a pocket pack of tissues
- One teaspoon butter or mayonnaise–a thimble, a thumb tip (top knuckle to tip), or the head of a toothbrush
- One ounce of cheese–your entire thumb, a tube of Chapstick, or an AA battery

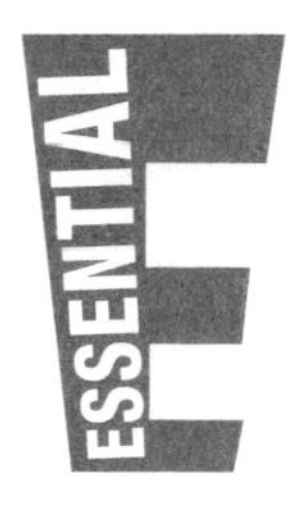

All-you-can-eat buffets are probably not the best choice for eating out. Americans like to feel as though they're getting a good deal on their meal; buffet restaurants try to capitalize on that sentiment by offering more dinner for your dollar, often at the expense of your waistline. If you really want to get your money's worth, get reacquainted with your kitchen.

Using your hands to estimate servings is probably the easiest method—you don't leave home without them. However, make sure you compare your hand amounts against food that has been measured out until you get a sense of how accurately you're estimating. Of course, if you have particularly large or small hands, you need to adjust for size.

Even for the more experienced portion predictor, it's a good idea to test your skills at least once a month and measure your guess at a serving size. It's easy to start overdoing it, and the little bits (and bites) add up. If your control has been off for no apparent reason, one of the first things to check is whether your serving sizes are on target.

Eating Out

Restaurants are notorious for serving up heaping helpings well beyond a single serving size. To keep your intake under control, you can split an entrée, order off the appetizer menu, or simply eat half and take half home. In some restaurants, you may be able to order a child-size portion (but even some children's menu items may be larger than a single serving). Ask your server to serve condiments on the side so your food isn't swimming in sauce, and stay away from the breadbasket, chips, or other complimentary snacks if you're fond of munching mindlessly.

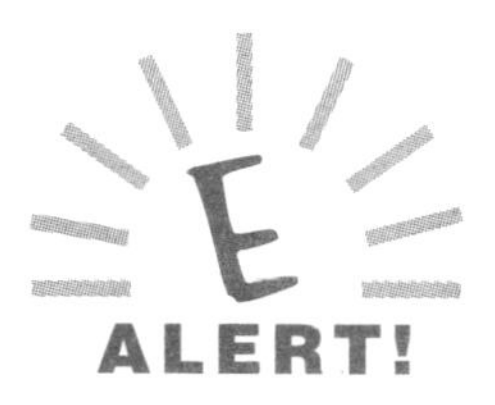

Many national restaurant chains, particularly fast-food establishments, will provide nutritional and serving size information on menu items upon request. Ask your server, or look online.

When planning a meal out, don't set yourself up for failure. Choose a place that you know offers some food choices that will fit in to your meal plan. If you must meet at the local greasy spoon where lard is a food group, fill up on a healthy meal at home first. If you're on the road or in unfamiliar territory, don't be afraid to phone first or ask to see a menu at the door before committing to a restaurant choice. Ask questions about ingredients and preparation method. If you feel a need to explain why you won't be eating somewhere, tell the hostess you're on a special diet. Some establishments may offer to prepare a dish in an alternate way (e.g., steaming instead of frying it) that isn't on the regular menu to keep your patronage.

When Temptation Strikes

You've had a delicious, yet healthy meal and are feeling pleased with yourself for turning down the bacon double cheeseburger that had been calling your name for broiled fish and steamed veggies. And then—the torture device rolls into view, a dessert cart laden with trays of your favorite cheesecake, hot fudge cake, and apple-caramel pie. You can feel your blood sugar rising just looking at it.

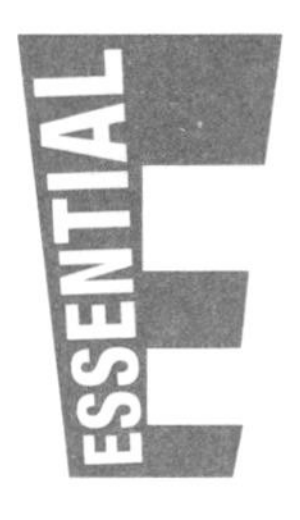

For some people, diabetes requires a major shift in their perception of food. If you see food as a reward system, a comfort when you're feeling down, or a symbol of love for your family, you need to develop positive replacements for it. Food is fuel—and while your tank will take a little sugar, look at the quantity and quality of what you're filling up on analytically rather than emotionally.

You can say "to hell with it!" and order the richest slab of carbs on the cart; grin and bear it while your dining companion savors his slice of pie à la mode; or use the situation as an opportunity to practice moderation. You will not be struck by lightning if you indulge occasionally, provided your splurges are factored in to your overall meal plan. Split a small dessert with a friend, or ask for half now and half in a takeout bag. If the offerings are truly too rich for your blood, promise yourself a frozen yogurt or another favorite treat on your way home. Don't deny yourself—it's not an all-or-nothing game. In fact, the stress of doing so constantly may raise your blood glucose levels higher than the occasional brownie.

Social occasions that are centered around eating, such as a birthday party, a holiday gathering, or a family reunion barbeque, offer a whole new set of challenges. Well-meaning friends and relatives frequently feel the need to be the food police, asking with every pass of the plate, "Should you be eating that?" The best answer is simple: "Most people with diabetes can eat just about anything you can, in moderation. I have a few books you can borrow that explain more if you're interested." Ideally, they'll take you up on your offer and learn a thing or two. If they don't, you've probably stopped them from pestering you, at least until Thanksgiving. Chapter 21 has more suggestions for handling food and special occasions.

Smart Snack Substitutes

Even though you can indulge occasionally, if you've made a regular habit of junk food, it's one you'll have to kick. Still, having many small meals, or minisnacks between meals, can be beneficial to keeping blood glucose on an even keel, and your RD will work these into your meal plan.

Cut out the fatty fried snacks, sugary drinks and sodas, and sugar-crusted snack pies, and try some of these healthier snack choices instead, all with around 15 grams of carbs (one carb choice) or less:

- Air-popped popcorn (3 cups)
- Snack-size sugar-free Jell-O with Cool Whip (both are considered free exchanges)
- Five whole-wheat crackers with peanut butter (1 tablespoon)
- Sugar-free pudding (½ cup)
- Two small tangerines
- Baked tortilla chips (15 to 20) and salsa

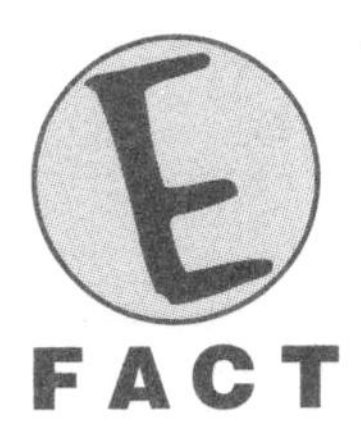

FACT

There are several types of meal bars on U.S. supermarket shelves formulated specifically for people with diabetes. Several are manufactured with cornstarch that has been processed in such a way that it breaks down very slowly in the digestive system, providing an even rise in blood glucose levels. Some people find these bars useful as a bedtime snack for warding off nighttime blood sugar lows.

Regaining Control After a Fall

If you haven't already, at one point in your life you will probably end up with an "Oh, Wow!" reading after splurging on something you shouldn't have. Ask yourself if there was a specific trigger for the slip-up, such as a particularly stressful day at work or going to a party hungry. If you can pinpoint a cause, think about how you can prevent it from happening next time, whether it be by adjusting your eating schedule or learning some stress management techniques.

It is not the end of the world if you screw up. If you're too busy kicking yourself, you'll miss any lesson you might gain from your mistake. Diabetes is a disease of highs and lows, both physically and emotionally. Strive to achieve balance in the emotional area as well as the physical one.

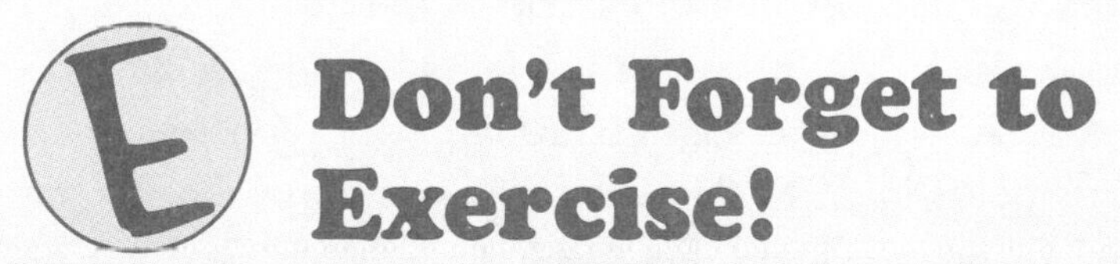

Chapter 12

Don't Forget to Exercise!

One of the simplest and most effective ways to bring down blood glucose levels, cut the risk of cardiovascular disease, and improve overall health and well-being is exercise. Yet in our increasingly sedentary world where almost every essential task can be performed online, from the driver's seat, or with a phone call, exercising can be a tough case to sell.

The Importance of Exercise

Everyone should exercise, yet the Surgeon General tells us that only 30 percent of the U.S. adult population gets the recommended thirty minutes of daily physical activity–and 25 percent aren't active at all. Inactivity is thought to be one of the key reasons for the surge of type 2 diabetes in America, because inactivity and obesity promote insulin resistance.

The good news is that it's never too late to get moving, and exercise is one of the easiest ways to start controlling your diabetes. For people with type 2 diabetes in particular, exercise can improve insulin sensitivity, lower the risk of heart disease, and promote weight loss.

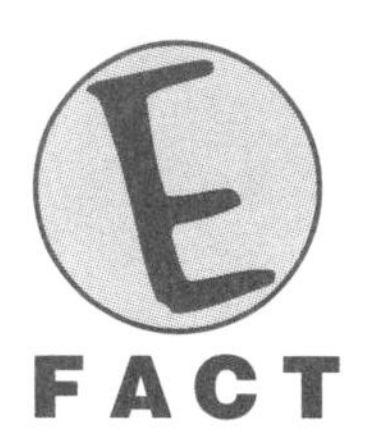

FACT

A 2003 animal study published in the *Journal of Clinical Endocrinology and Metabolism* found that lack of exercise—and not diet—were the key factors behind obesity and diabetes. The findings suggest that exercise may play an even bigger role than previously thought in diabetes control and prevention in humans.

While several studies have demonstrated that regular exercise can lower A1c (average long-term glucose) levels in type 2 diabetes, more research is needed to firmly establish that link. As of early 2003, there was no clinical data supporting a long-term A1c-lowering effect in type 1 diabetes. But despite the lack of conclusive scientific evidence at this point in time, exercise still has many benefits for people with type 1 diabetes, including improved blood cholesterol levels, lower blood pressure, better heart health, and the short-term suppression of blood glucose levels.

Getting Started

The first order of business with any exercise plan, especially if you're a dyed-in-the-wool couch potato, is to consult with your health care provider. If you have cardiac risk factors, she may want to perform a stress test to establish a safe level of exercise for you.

Certain diabetic complications will also dictate what type of exercise program you can take on. Activities like weightlifting, jogging, or high-impact aerobics can possibly pose a risk for people with diabetic retinopathy due to the risk for further blood vessel damage and possible retinal detachment. And the ADA recommends that patients with severe peripheral neuropathy (PN) avoid foot-intensive weight-bearing exercises such as long-distance walking, jogging, or step aerobics and opt instead for low-impact activities like swimming, biking, and rowing. If you have conditions that make exercise a challenge, your provider may refer you to an exercise physiologist who can design a fitness program for your specific needs.

If you're already active in sports or work out regularly, it will still benefit you to discuss your regular routine with your doctor. If you're taking insulin, you may need to take special precautions to prevent hypoglycemia during your workout.

Start Slow

Your exercise routine can be as simple as a brisk nightly neighborhood walk. If you haven't been very active before now, start slowly and work your way up. Walk the dog or get out in the yard and rake. Take the stairs instead of the elevator. Park in the back of the lot and walk. Every little bit does, in fact, help.

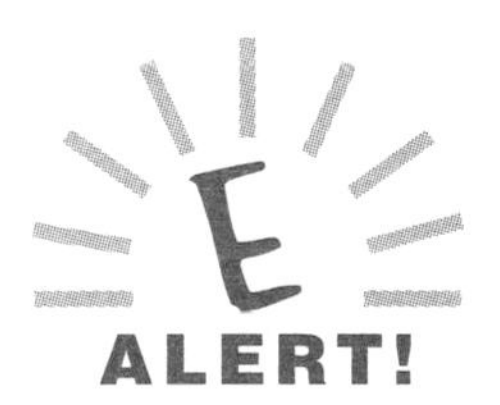

Leg pain during exercise, especially aching in the calves, buttocks, or thighs, could be intermittent claudication and peripheral vascular disease (a potential complication of diabetes). Physician-supervised exercise, particularly walking, can actually help ease the pain over time. Medication may also be required.

As little as fifteen to thirty minutes of daily, heart-pumping exercise can make a big difference in your blood glucose control and your risk of developing diabetic complications. One of the easiest and least expensive ways of getting moving is to start a walking program. All you need is a good pair of well-fitting, supportive shoes and a direction to head in.

Do pay particular attention to your feet both before and after you walk or run. Because of the risk for foot ulcers and other diabetic foot problems, you should examine them carefully for blisters and abrasions and treat them promptly if they do occur. Seamless, waterproof socks that wick moisture away from your feet can help to prevent friction while walking. For more on diabetic foot care, see Chapter 16.

Making Time

Everyone is busy. But considering what's at stake, making time for exercise needs to be a priority right now. Thirty minutes a day isn't much when you get right down to it. Cut one prime-time show out of your evening television viewing schedule. Get up a half-hour earlier each morning. Use half of your lunch hour for a brisk walk. You can find the time if you look hard enough for it.

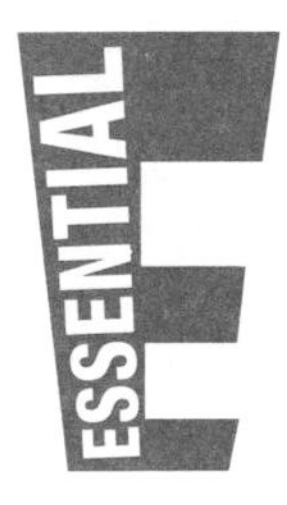

You don't have to spend a lot of money on expensive health club memberships, treadmills, or the latest fitness gadget to get moving. However, some people find that if they make a monetary investment, they're more likely to follow through on fitness. If you don't have a lot of money to spend, investigate a basic membership at your local YMCA, YWCA, or community center.

You can also try combining exercise with something else already on your schedule. If you normally spend an hour on Saturday morning playing video games with your kids, take it out of virtual reality and play a real game of touch football or Frisbee outside. Get off the riding mower and cut the grass the old-fashioned way—with a manual push mower. Wake up early and walk your kids to school. Look for opportunities rather than excuses.

Exercise Intensity

How hard you should be pushing yourself depends on your level of fitness and your health history. Your doctor can recommend an optimal heart rate target for working out based on these factors.

On average, most people should aim for a target heart rate zone of 50 to 75 percent of your maximum heart rate. Maximum heart rate is computed by subtracting your age from the number 220. So if you are 40, your maximum heart rate would be 180, and your target heart rate zone would be between 90 and 135 beats per minute.

You should wear a digital or analog watch with a second hand or function to check your heart rate during exercise. You can calculate heart rate by placing your fingers at your wrist or neck pulse point and counting the number of beats for fifteen seconds. Multiply that number by four to get your heart rate.

The number you get should be within your target zone. If it's too high, take your intensity down a few notches. If you're exercising below your target zone, pick things up. If you are new to exercise, you should aim for the lower (50 percent) range of your target heart rate. As you become more fit, you can work toward the 75 percent maximum.

Blood Sugars and Exercise

When you exercise, your body uses glucose for energy. During the first fifteen minutes of your workout routine, your body converts the glycogen stored in your muscles back into glucose, and also uses the glucose circulating in your bloodstream for fuel. This action causes the natural blood-glucose-lowering effect of exercise.

After fifteen minutes, your body turns to the liver to convert its glycogen stockpile into glucose energy. After about thirty minutes, your cells will also begin to burn free fatty acids (FFA) for fuel. Once the glycogen stores are used up, without a carb refueling in the form of food, hypoglycemia is a real danger, particularly to those with type 1 diabetes.

Before you get moving, test your glucose levels. If they are less than 100 mg/dl, don't start working out without a carbohydrate snack for fuel. A fast-acting carb should be available during and after your workout, in case you need it.

Snacking Savvy

Because of the risk of hypoglycemia during exercise, especially in type 1 diabetes, a pre-exercise snack may be required. How much of a snack and when to eat it depends on your blood glucose readings and the planned intensity and duration of your workout. In general, people with type 2 diabetes who work out at a moderate level will probably not require a snack before exercise, particularly if they are trying to lose weight.

For people with type 1 diabetes, moderately intense exercise lasting longer than a half-hour will probably require a snack of at least 15 grams of carbohydrates. If you're planning on a high-energy game of racquetball that may last an hour or more, you will need a bigger carb boost of between 25 to 50 grams of carbohydrates. Adding protein and/or fat to the carbs can extend the glucose action over time if you're embarking on a long-distance bike ride or similar activity. A snack should be taken about fifteen to thirty minutes before exercise for the best results.

If you're going on a low-intensity, half-hour walk and your glucose readings are at least 100 mg/dl, you may not need any extra carbs (although you should always bring some with you just in case).

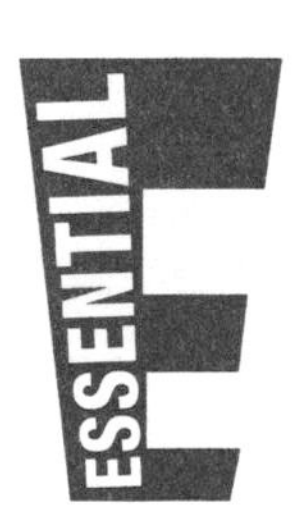

Keeping an exercise log along with your blood glucose readings can help you figure out what works best for you. Different sports and routines will have diverse effects on your blood sugar levels. Discuss your exercise plans with your diabetes care team to find out the best routine for preparing for exercise.

Never exercise immediately following a regular meal. Give your body time—at least ninety minutes—to digest and process injected insulin. Don't plan exercise during the time your insulin is peaking. Exercise can also cause injected insulin to work much faster because your circulation is speeded up as your heart pumps harder. In many cases, you may need to adjust your insulin dose downward for those times you will be exercising; again, your doctor can offer you further advice on what's right for you.

Lows (Hypoglycemia)

If you start to feel hypoglycemia coming on, don't panic. Stop exercising and test immediately. If your levels are too low, eat or drink 15 grams of carbohydrate right away. Don't resume your workout. Wait fifteen minutes for the carbs to kick in and test again. If your levels are still too low, take 15 more grams and follow the same routine until blood glucose levels are back in a normal range.

A glucose gel or glucose tablet is a good choice for a fast-acting carb. Both are compact enough to carry along while you exercise and work quickly. Invest in a waterproof fanny pack to keep both your glucose gel/tablets and testing supplies in during your workout.

After your workout is finished, your body will recharge its energy stores by processing your blood glucose into glycogen. Depending on the level of exercise intensity and the amount of glycogen that needs to be replaced, this process could take anywhere from four to twenty-four hours. This is why postexercise glucose testing is important, as hypoglycemia can occur well after you've finished exercising.

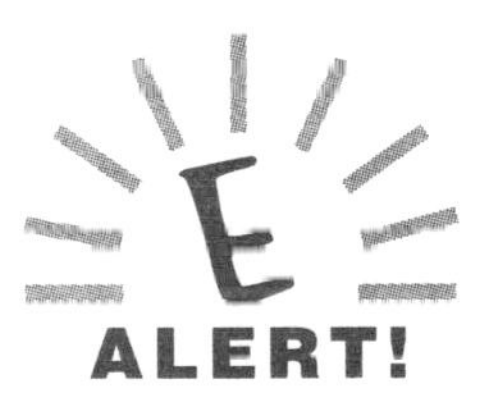

The ADA suggests that people with type 1 diabetes temporarily avoid physical activity if fasting glucose levels are greater than 250 mg/dl and ketosis is present, and use caution if glucose levels are greater than 300 mg/dl and no ketosis is present.

Highs (Hyperglycemia)

In some cases, when blood glucose levels are high and insulin levels are low to begin with, the adrenaline rush from heavy exercise can have the opposite affect, signaling the liver and muscles to break down glycogen into glucose. In these cases, ketoacidosis is a danger. If your blood sugars test high before exercise, *always* test for ketones before you start your workout. If your levels are high and you do choose to exercise, make sure you test glucose levels again about fifteen minutes into your workout to ensure they are coming back down.

Take Precautions

To avoid dangerous highs and lows during exercise, take the following precautions:

- **Test first.** Always take a blood glucose reading before your workout.
- **Warm up.** Always stretch out before exercising to avoid injury, and start your routine with five to ten minutes of low-intensity movement.
- **Wet down.** Drink plenty of fluids before, during, and after your workout to prevent dehydration. If you're exercising in the heat, drink even more.
- **Cool off.** If you're working out intensely, take it down a few notches at a time, and spend five to ten minutes bringing your heart rate back down to its preworkout level.
- **Carb load.** Have a fast-acting carbohydrate on hand in case of hypoglycemia, and don't hesitate to use it.
- **Test last.** Once your workout is over, test your blood glucose levels again to ensure they aren't dipping too low.

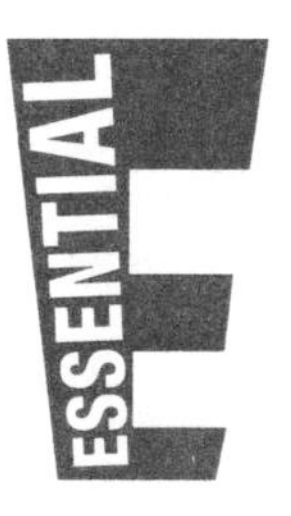

You should always wear or carry medical identification, but it's particularly important when you are exercising. Before you go for that run, make sure you are wearing your ID in a visible location. A shoelace tag or watchband ID are sports-friendly options if you find your regular ID bracelet or necklace gets in the way of your workout.

Everyone Can Exercise

Virtually everyone who has the capability to move can exercise to some degree. Even if you suffer from complications related to your diabetes or other health conditions, your doctor can recommend a level and form of exercise that is appropriate for you.

Chances are that you already work out without even knowing it. Things you have never considered "exercise," like washing the car or cleaning your house, are actually calorie-burning, heart-pumping ways to get fit. According to the U.S. Surgeon General, all of the following activities will burn about 150 calories a day (or 1,000 calories a week):

- Washing and waxing a car for 45 to 60 minutes
- Washing windows or floors for 45 to 60 minutes
- Gardening for 30 to 45 minutes
- Pushing a stroller 1.5 miles in 30 minutes
- Raking leaves for 30 minutes
- Walking 2 miles in 30 minutes (15 minutes per mile)
- Doing water aerobics for 30 minutes
- Bicycling 4 miles in 15 minutes
- Shoveling snow for 15 minutes
- Climbing steps for 15 minutes

Disabled and Chronically Ill

For people with orthopedic conditions, joint pain, or musculoskeletal problems, low-impact exercise is usually the best bet. Swimming is a good low-impact form of resistance exercise. If you are in a wheelchair or unable to stand or stay on your feet for long periods of time without support, chair exercises may also be a good option. There are a number of chair exercise videotapes available for home workouts.

Dealing with Obesity

If you are extremely overweight or obese, exercise is especially important, yet can present unique challenges. Comfort is an issue; certain exercises like jogging and high-impact aerobics may simply not be feasible. Weight lies heavy on the mind as well as the body, and it's possible you may not be feeling mentally or emotionally prepared to join group or team exercises.

Work on your own level. Don't try step aerobics just yet. Contact your local Y or community center to see if there's a plus-size exercise program available. And always check with your doctor before starting a new fitness routine. A referral to an exercise physiologist may be appropriate, particularly if you have other health problems.

It may be easier said than done, but don't feel self-conscious. If you feel uncomfortable amid all the spandex and ripped abs at the local health club, then don't torture yourself—find an environment that you feel at ease in. Try a walking program, either outside or at home on a treadmill. The impact-free environment of a pool is also a good place to start getting fit. Buddy up with a friend and motivate each other. Exercise should make you feel good about yourself. Every step you take is a step toward a healthier you.

Exercising for the Elderly

Staying active is particularly important as you grow older. Aging is associated with increased insulin resistance, and it's thought that this is at least partially attributable to a loss of muscle mass. Keep on track with an active lifestyle and strength-training exercises to retain muscle mass and insulin sensitivity. It's never too late to get moving. Talk to your doctor today about an appropriate exercise program that promotes strength, balance, flexibility, and endurance.

Get Your Kids to Exercise, Too

Children with type 1 diabetes are probably the least likely to need motivation to exercise. After all, most parents have a harder time keeping kids quiet than getting them moving. Yet because of often unpredictable blood glucose levels, particularly in younger children, they also are the group that probably requires the most vigilance in monitoring to avoid exercise-induced hypoglycemia. They also play hard, so testing should be frequent even in the absence of structured sports or exercise.

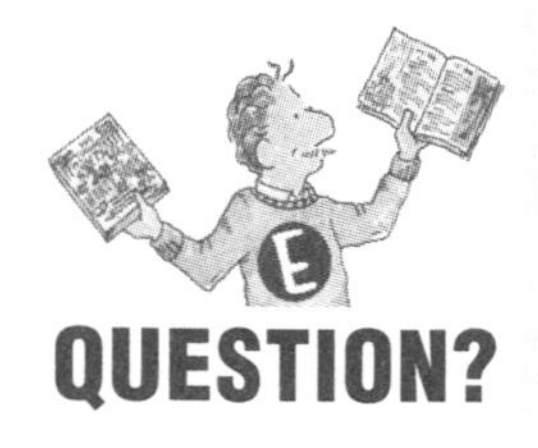

My daughter has type 1 diabetes and wants to join a soccer team. Should I let her?

By all means! Children with diabetes should be encouraged to take part in the same activities as their peers. However, coaches and other adults that oversee your child's participation in team or individual sports should be educated about the signs and treatment of hypoglycemia.

For overweight children or adolescents with type 2 diabetes, or those who are considered at risk for the disease, exercise is absolutely imperative for all the reasons previously cited for adults—weight loss, improved insulin sensitivity, and overall health and well-being.

Staying Motivated

One of the biggest obstacles to staying on track for fitness is losing motivation. People who are just starting an exercise program can find themselves quickly tired of the same routine. Keeping exercise appealing and maintaining a good fitness perspective is key to long-term success.

Boredom Busters

If you had to watch the exact same episode of your favorite television show every day for the rest of your life, you'd probably be banging your head against the wall by the end of the week. You'd change the channel, pick up a book, or do anything you could to avoid something you once enjoyed. Yet many people starting on a fitness program feel compelled to follow the same routine, day after day after day, and consequently fall off the exercise wagon due to sheer boredom. Try these strategies for keeping your workouts interesting.

- **Mix and match.** Play racquetball with a friend one week and try water polo the next.
- **Buddy up.** Get a walking partner or an exercise buddy to keep you motivated (and vice versa).
- **Join a team.** Find a local softball league or aerobics group. Even when you aren't feeling much like exercising, your commitment to other team members may get you moving.
- **Relocate.** If you like to bike, walk, or jog, try a new route or locale.
- **Go for the goal.** Set new fitness targets for yourself.
- **Reward yourself.** When you reach a new goal, pat yourself on the back with a nonedible reward.
- **Make some noise.** Forget the radio and your CDs and customize your own soundtrack for working out.

- **Be well read.** Exercise your mind as well as your body with an audiobook.
- **Sound off.** Try it without the Walkman for once, and enjoy the sounds of nature and the neighborhood.

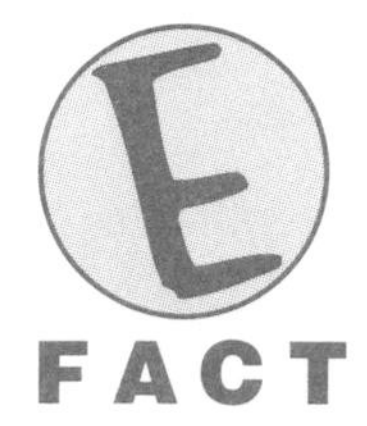

FACT

If you or someone you know is at risk for developing type 2 diabetes, getting fit can help. The Diabetes Prevention Trial found that minor lifestyle changes, including just thirty minutes of exercise daily, cut the risk of developing type 2 diabetes in high-risk subjects by 58 percent.

Keeping It in Perspective

Many people, particularly those with type 2 diabetes, start exercising for the sole purpose of losing weight. When the pounds don't drop as quickly or as completely as they'd like, they get discouraged and give up. If you take away any message about exercise and diabetes, let it be this: Even if you don't lose weight, your investment in exercise is still paying off in reduced heart disease risk and better blood glucose control. And exercise simply makes you feel better, both physically and mentally. Your energy level will rise and the endorphins released by your brain during exercise will boost your sense of well-being and may help fight diabetes-related depression. Don't give up before you really get started. You owe it to yourself to keep going.

Athletes and Athletics

What do Olympic Gold Medalist Gary Hall Jr., NBA athlete Chris Dudley, LPGA golfer Kelli Kuehne, and NFL player Mike Echols all have in common? They have all successfully managed to balance type 1 diabetes with high-performance athletics, no small accomplishment given everything you've just learned about insulin, exercise, and blood glucose control.

Outside of a pie-eating contest, there is virtually no competitive event that well-controlled type 1 or type 2 diabetes can exclude you from. But athletes with diabetes must have exemplary self-management skills and be very attuned to their reactions to different levels of activity. They must be as dedicated to blood glucose control as they are to their sport of choice.

Team sports in particular require a coaching staff and team members who are flexible about treatment breaks for blood glucose checks and other essentials. For the most successful relationship, team members and leaders should also be educated about the needs of athletes with diabetes and the signs and treatment of a hypo episode.

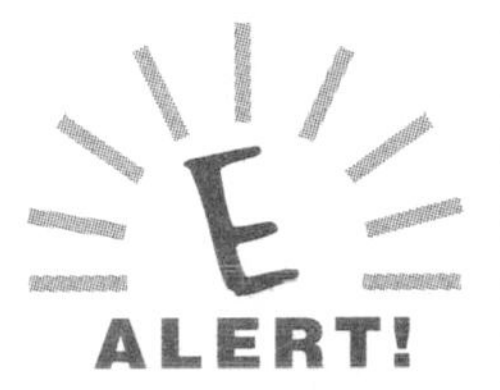

Even a mild episode of hypoglycemia could have lethal consequences in some high-risk sports like scuba diving or rock climbing. Athletes who choose to participate in sports that demand a high level of concentration need to have a partner familiar with the symptoms of a blood sugar low to ensure safety.

Whether your goal is professional athletics or just a friendly pickup game at the park, working closely with your health care team and remaining aware of the signals your body sends is the best way to attain it.

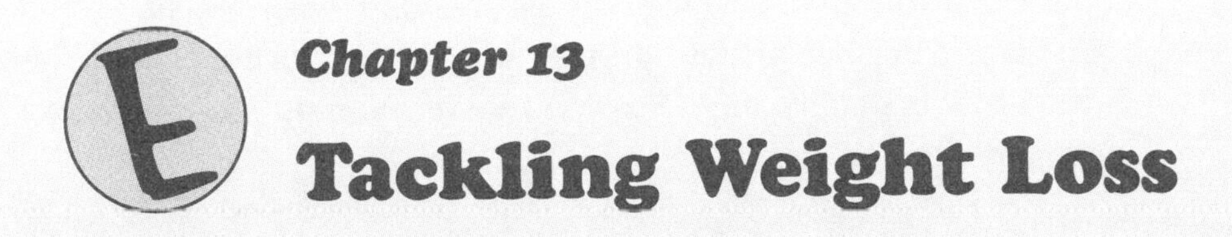

Chapter 13

Tackling Weight Loss

Up to 90 percent of people with type 2 diabetes are overweight. In fact, America as a nation has been packing on the pounds for the past two decades, with a whopping one-third of all adults classified as obese and skyrocketing rates of childhood obesity. Losing weight is one of the best ways to treat type 2 diabetes, but it is also possibly the most difficult. And people with type 1 diabetes have to deal with special insulin-related weight problems of their own.

In Control and Gaining Weight

People with type 1 diabetes face a unique challenge with weight. Frequently, when they start getting their blood glucose levels under control with insulin injections, their weight goes up. When blood sugars are high, your body becomes dehydrated, and as your blood sugars come under control and your fluid balance returns, you gain water weight.

This is actually a positive development when it occurs shortly after diagnosis; this weight gain helps you recover pounds you may have lost leading up to diagnosis.

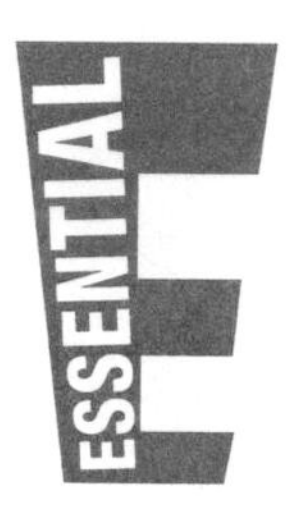

Better control sometimes comes at the cost of a few extra pounds. The Diabetes Control and Complications Trial (DCCT) found that as blood glucose levels in type 1 diabetes came down to normal levels, subjects gained an average of 10 pounds.

The Role of Insulin

Injected insulin is also helping your body to utilize glucose energy from food. Before you started treatment for your type 1 diabetes, you may have found that you could eat virtually anything to try to quiet your ravenous hyperglycemia-induced appetite, and you would not gain a pound. Now that you actually have the insulin to help process the glucose, you'll gain weight, a sign that you're also gaining control over your diabetes. It may also take a while for you to get your appetite back in sync with your newfound control, which can also cause extra weight gain.

Don't get too discouraged by weight gain that occurs with the start of insulin treatment. Again, it's usually a sign you're getting better, not bigger. If you continue to gain weight or become concerned about the weight you've gained so far, a strategy session with your doctor and dietitian is in order. They may be able to recommend dietary and insulin adjustments that can help bring unwanted weight gain to a halt. Sometimes a switch to a different insulin type or an insulin pump can help you to get a handle on weight fluctuations.

Type 2 and Insulin

People with type 2 diabetes who switch to insulin injections to achieve better control over their blood sugars can also find themselves gaining weight. If you are type 2 and are already overweight or obese, weight gain can increase your insulin resistance, which in turn will increase your insulin dose requirement. It's essential to talk to your doctor about possible adjustments to treatment before you find yourself in a vicious cycle of insulin resistance and weight gain.

Type 2 Medications and Weight Gain

Some of the hypoglycemic drugs prescribed for type 2 diabetes can cause weight gain as well. Insulin-sensitizing thiazolidinediones (also called TZDs or glitizones), including Actos (pioglitazone) and Avandia (rosiglitazone), and sulfonylurea drugs fall into this category. Because TZDs can also cause edema, weight gain from their use may mean a gain in fluids rather than fat.

On the flip side, metformin can cause weight loss in some people. If you're taking one of these drugs, your doctor may add metformin to the mix if you're experiencing weight gain as a side effect. Combination drugs can eliminate the need for two prescription drugs. For Avandia users, the combination drug Avandamet (rosiglitazone and metformin) may be prescribed; DiaBeta, Glynase, and Micronase users may benefit from Glucovance (glyburide and metformin); and Glucotrol users may be prescribed Metaglip (glipizide and metformin). Combination drugs are not an option for all type 2 patients. Talk to your doctor about whether or not they may be right for you.

Weight Loss and Type 2 Diabetes

The Diabetes Prevention Program (DPP) proved that even modest weight loss can prevent or delay the onset of type 2 diabetes in overweight at-risk adults. But what about people who already have the disease? The news is good for you as well. Weight loss can reduce your need for medication and insulin, improve your cardiovascular health, and, best of all, it will make you feel good about yourself.

Weight and Insulin Resistance

Precisely how excess fat promotes insulin resistance isn't yet entirely clear, but it is thought that certain proteins and/or enzymes released by stored fat act on muscle and liver cells to impair the way that they "read" insulin signals to process glucose.

In addition, research has found that the "apple-shaped" body (central abdominal obesity) associated with insulin resistance and type 2 diabetes contains fat with unique properties. Specifically, this type of visceral abdominal fat sheds more free fatty acids, which can elevate triglyceride levels, and is associated with higher insulin levels that promote further fat storage. Paring down your abdominal fat has the double benefit of both increasing insulin sensitivity and decreasing triglyceride levels in people with type 2 diabetes.

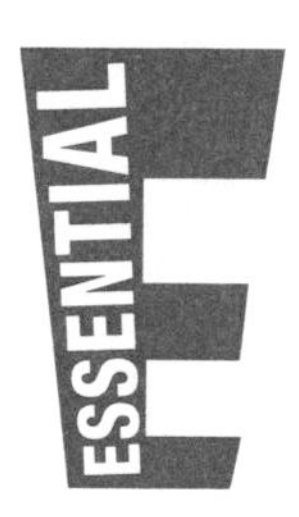

Among American adults, women are more likely to be obese than men (33 percent compared to 28 percent). African-American and Mexican-American women, who are already at greater risk for developing type 2 diabetes, have some of the highest rates of obesity (50 and 40 percent, respectively).

Shedding Smart

First and foremost, you need a plan that dovetails with your diabetes management program. Book a date with your dietitian so you can strategize on meal plans to promote weight loss. Talk to your doctor before embarking on any new exercise plan so he can assess your heart health and give your workout his official stamp of approval.

If you have diabetic complications or other health issues that affect your mobility, an exercise physiologist and/or physical therapist may be able to get you on track with a low-impact or adaptive exercise program.

Set Realistic Goals

Many people end up abandoning perfectly good weight-loss programs before they even lace up their sneakers. Why? Because in a world filled with fast food, instant messaging, and five-second glucose meters, anything without a quick payoff goes against the grain of the American instant gratification ethic. While it would be nice to "drop inches in days!" like the miracle ads proclaim, weight loss is a slow and (hopefully) steady process that takes time and commitment.

Setting weight-loss goals for yourself can be a good motivator. Gradual weight loss is usually the safest. A diet that cuts your normal calorie consumption (for your weight) by 500 to 1,000 per day will encourage weight loss. So will burning 500 to 1,000 calories each day with exercise. Your best bet is to strike a balance between the two, and make exercise—be it team sports, cycling, or walking—something you enjoy. Making a long-term healthy lifestyle change is essential to keeping the pounds off once they're gone.

Aim Low

If you wear a size 14 and you blow a bundle on a designer size 8 dress as motivation, you'll probably end up feeling guilty, frustrated, and angry if you aren't slinking around in it a month later. You'll do much better setting smaller, achievable targets for yourself. If you must try the new-clothes strategy, go down a size at a time, and don't buy anything you have to take out a second mortgage to pay for.

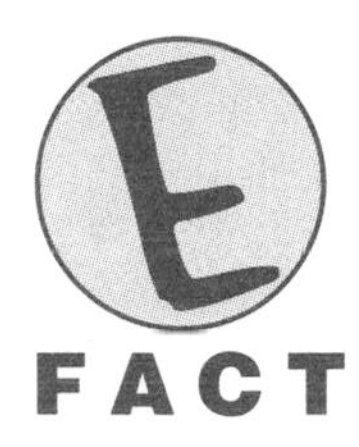

An estimated 5.3 million, or 12.5 percent, of Americans between ages six and seventeen are obese. Childhood obesity has led to an alarming increase in type 2 diabetes, once considered an "adults-only" disease, and can lead to a variety of other weight-related medical problems later in life.

Because weight loss can be a long and bumpy road, you'll find your enthusiasm waning occasionally. Try these strategies to stay inspired and on track.

- **Compete and commiserate.** Set weight-loss goals along with a friend or spouse. A little friendly competition can be just the motivation you need, and you'll also have someone to call to talk you down when that ice cream sundae just won't stop calling your name.
- **Reward yourself.** Find nonedible indulgences to tell yourself "good job!"
- **Scale back.** Don't weigh yourself obsessively. Once a week–at the same time of day–is all you need to keep tabs on your progress.
- **Take baby steps.** Everyone starts somewhere. Even a walk around the block is better than sitting on the couch wishing you had the stamina to go on a bike ride with your kids.

Need more motivation? See Chapter 12 for ways to keep exercise interesting.

What Doesn't Work

There are also plenty of weight-loss strategies that are guaranteed to backfire:

- **Skipping meals.** Forgoing food completely is hard on your diabetes control, may cause a hypo, and will probably only be effective in making you eat twice as much at the next meal.
- **Skipping meds.** Purposely skipping your shots is spinning the DKA roulette wheel. Insulin omission is not an effective method of weight loss and can trigger dangerous highs.
- **Dieting without exercise, or vice versa.** Decreasing calories and increasing activity are both required for successful weight loss.
- **Perpetual procrastination.** Waiting for a "better time" to start a weight-loss plan won't make it any easier, and it can quite possibly make the task harder. Stop waiting for tomorrow, and begin today.

Mind over Matter

Losing weight with diabetes means you have two challenges to conquer–learning what and how to eat for optimal blood glucose control, and breaking away from bad overeating habits.

Eating emotionally rather than in response to hunger cues is at the root of many weight problems. Examine what your "eating triggers" are. Do you use food as a reward, a comfort, a social tool, or simply a release from boredom? The first step in breaking these habits is recognizing them, and then coming up with positive substitutions.

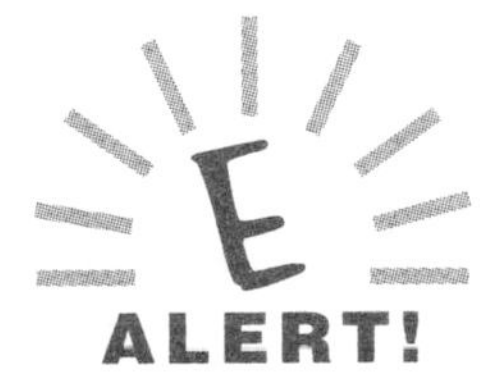

Try to rely more on the way you feel than the tale of the tape. If the scale tells you you're losing weight slower than you'd like, but you're feeling energetic and positive about your weight-loss efforts, then you're doing fine. Again, weight loss is not a quick process.

Make a reward something that feeds your soul rather than your stomach—a few hours with a good book or a weekend getaway with someone special. Try to come up with ways to socialize that aren't focused on food. Meet at a coffeehouse rather than a restaurant, or meet up to play football or Frisbee rather than spending another afternoon as armchair quarterbacks.

Above all, practice mindful eating. Have meals and snacks away from the television and other distractions that make it too easy to gobble up twice as much as you intended to. Enjoy your food, and then move on. Fortunately, good diabetes management encourages mindful eating.

The Low-Carb Conundrum

Low-carb diets are the subject of heated debate in the diabetes community. At first glance, the issue seems cut-and-dried. Carbohydrates cause glucose to rise, so wouldn't a low-carb diet automatically be beneficial for someone with diabetes? But low-carb also turns the traditional food pyramid on its head, and goes against everything the USDA and nutritionists have been saying for the past several decades—that the vast majority of your calories (50 to 60 percent) should come from carbohydrates.

In a nutshell, low-carb proponents blame weight gain on high insulin levels, which can promote fat storage. Since insulin release is triggered by dietary carbohydrates, the reasoning is that too many carbs means too much glucose, which in turn leads to high levels of insulin, which cause fat storage and weight gain.

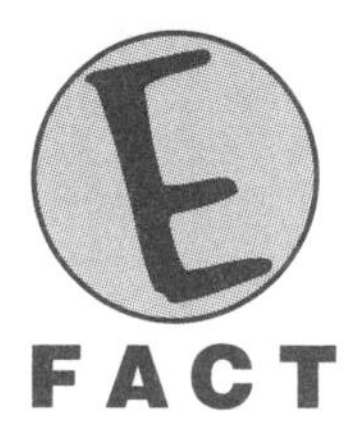

FACT

One of the most popular low-carb plans was created by Dr. Richard Bernstein, who has type 1 diabetes and helped to pioneer the concept of regular self-monitoring of blood glucose levels. The plan is described in his book, *Dr. Bernstein's Diabetes Solution* (Little, Brown & Company, 1997).

The Risks Involved

The ADA does not endorse Atkins and similar low-carb plans, saying that the high-fat and high-protein content in these diets can be dangerous for people with diabetes who are already at risk for coronary artery disease. The other problem with low-carb diets is that the high-protein content can be tough on the kidneys of people who have any degree of renal impairment. The Atkins Center itself says that anyone with severe kidney disease (described as a creatinine level of 2.4 or higher) should not do the program.

That said, there are many people who swear by them—saying that low-carbing has given them their blood sugar control back. Most successful low-carbing involves attention to calories as well as carbs; too much fat can add too many calories to your diet, and without calorie reduction weight loss simply won't occur. If you do decide to give low-carb dieting a try, discuss it with your doctor first, and work with your RD on a customized plan for you.

The issue of the safety of low-carb approaches was high profile enough to warrant a 2000 USDA-sponsored roundtable called "The Great Nutrition Debate," which pitted low-carb luminaries, including the late Dr. Atkins, against pyramid proponents and other nutritional gurus. Although the conference didn't have any far-reaching policy implications, it did reveal the growing dichotomy between the nutrition establishment and low-carbohydrate advocates.

In May 2003, the *New England Journal of Medicine* published two controlled trials that put low-carb to the test among people with significant weight and health problems. One study found that obese participants with diabetes who were restricted to 30 grams of carbs daily achieved greater weight loss, maintained better glucose control, and cut triglyceride levels more than their counterparts who were put on a low-fat diet. The second trial had a smaller study population but came to similar conclusions. However, the authors also concluded that the difference in these health benefits between low-fat and low-carb became insignificant after the first six months. Further long-term, large-scale trials are needed to analyze the risks and potential pluses of low-carb in diabetes treatment.

Glycemic Index Diets

And then there's the glycemic index, the subject of many bestselling diet books–i.e., *Sugar Busters* (Ballantine) and *The Glucose Revolution*– and another dietary hot potato. The GI focuses on the choice of carbs rather than carb restriction. Low-GI foods raise blood glucose levels at a slow and steady rate, promoting weight loss by discouraging blood sugar spikes and high circulating levels of insulin. The GI has a solid foundation in science and many faithful followers, but requires some dedicated math skills and an even more dedicated patient. For more on the glycemic index, see Chapter 11.

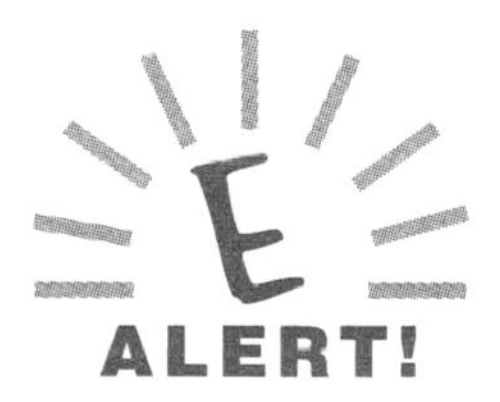

Most fad diets are just that—a fleeting fancy. At best, they drain your wallet and your self-confidence; at their worst, they can be hazardous to your health. Anything that claims dramatic results in days or a few weeks, that relies on "testimonials" instead of hard science, or that uses lots of buzzwords to cover up a serious lack of substance is probably destined for failure.

Drugs and Surgery

When diet and exercise just aren't doing the job for whatever reason, there are other options. Some weight-loss medications such as Xenical (orlistat) may have some promise in treating obesity. In clinical trials,

Xenical produced a 5 percent or higher weight loss in 72 percent of subjects over a period of six months. The mean weight loss was 23 pounds. The ADA recommends that weight-loss medications only be used in patients with a BMI of 27 or higher, and always in conjunction with lifestyle modifications (i.e., diet and exercise).

Bariatric Surgery

Finally, for severely obese people with type 2 diabetes who have been unable to lose weight using traditional means, gastric bypass or reduction surgery may be an option. Only patients with a BMI greater than or equal to 35 are typically considered for bariatric surgery.

There are a number of different types of bariatric surgery, including adjustable gastric banding, vertical banded gastroplasty, Roux-en-Y gastric bypass, and biliopancreatic diversion (with or without a duodenal switch). The first two of these are restrictive surgeries, and work by closing off the majority of the stomach to the digestive process, leaving only a small section to digest food. The latter two are bypass (or malabsorptive) operations, which reroute the digestive flow past part or all of the small intestine to minimize the amount of calories absorbed.

Bariatric surgery carries the same risks of infection and hemorrhage as any major surgery, plus a high rate of related complications; up to 20 percent of people who have bariatric surgery have to undergo a follow-up operation to fix abdominal hernia or other problems. Gallstones are also a risk because of the rapid weight loss that occurs following the operation.

And because some types of surgery bypass the small intestine, where a great deal of nutrient absorption takes place, approximately 30 percent of patients end up with deficiencies of certain vitamins and minerals (a condition that can usually be corrected with supplementation).

Keeping It Off

Weight maintenance can be a lifelong challenge. Sometimes you can't control the situations that put the pounds back on. Illness or injury can hamper your exercise efforts, or required drug therapy may promote weight gain. When health conditions cause weight gain, sometimes the only thing you can do is wait it out and get back on your program when things resolve.

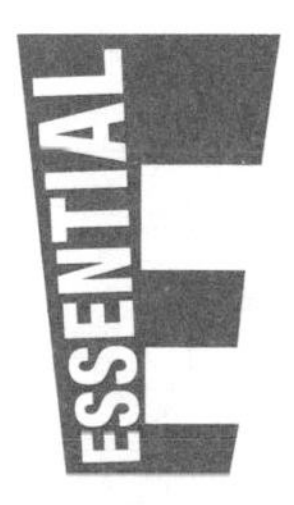

Keep a diary of your weight-loss progress—it can help you become familiar with the things that trigger weight gain and slip-ups for you, and make you much less likely to fall prey to them next time around.

But slipping back into old habits like emotional eating, exercise avoidance, or plain old procrastination can be avoided. In fact, having diabetes may make it easier to stay on track, since you have to pay attention to your body by default. And when you do stumble, remember that it isn't the end of the world. You're simply learning another lesson about yourself and your health that will benefit your emotional management of diabetes in the long run.

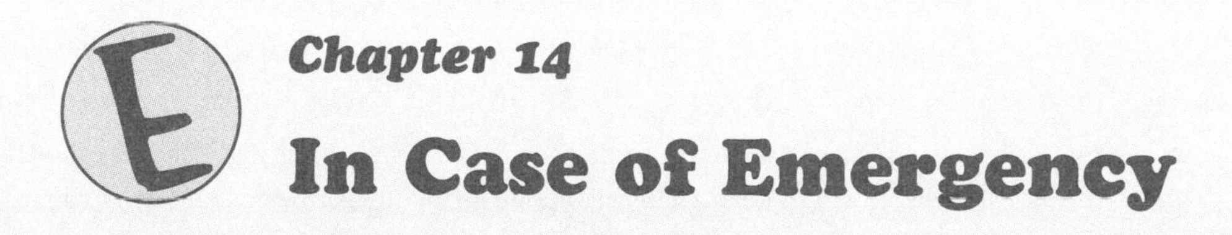

Chapter 14

In Case of Emergency

One minute you're fine, the next you are dizzy, shaky, and disoriented. Blood sugar highs and lows—the literal peaks and valleys of diabetes—are perhaps the scariest part of the disease. Preparation, prevention, and patience are the keys to getting through them and staying in control of your diabetes.

Hypoglycemic Episodes

Hypoglycemia, also called an insulin reaction, blood sugar low, or a hypo, can hit hard and fast. If you have type 1 diabetes, you are more likely to experience blood glucose lows than if you have type 2 diabetes (although people with type 2 can experience hypos as well).

What exactly constitutes a low varies from person to person. Everyone has differing levels of sensitivity to blood glucose drops. One person may start to feel "funny" at 70 mg/dl (3.9 mmol/l), while another can drop considerably lower before sensing something is wrong. Still others suffer from a condition known as *hypoglycemic unawareness*, in which the body no longer reacts to low blood glucose levels with the usual symptoms. Your doctor will help you establish what reading is too low for you.

Low episodes are typically caused by one of three things:

1. Too much insulin or diabetes medication (sulfonylureas or meglitinides)
2. Too little food
3. Exercise without enough carbohydrates

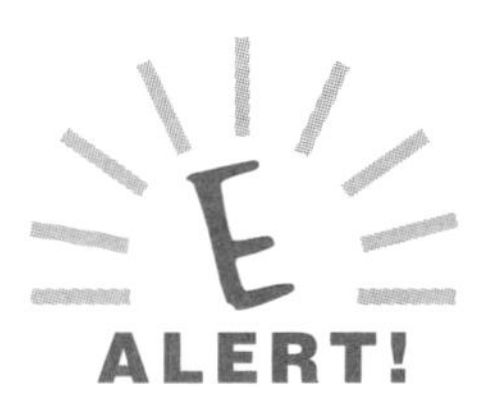

Exercise naturally lowers blood glucose levels, so if you're working out, you should test before, during (about a half-hour in), and after exercising. For more on exercise and diabetes, see Chapter 12.

When it comes to dealing effectively with hypoglycemia, you need to be prepared, practice prevention, and exercise patience. Carry a fast-acting sugar or carb at all times; test often and treat at the first sign of a low; and don't panic and down 2 liters of soda, or you can easily end up on a roller coaster of highs and lows.

Signs and Symptoms

Blood sugar lows are dangerous because the central nervous system needs glucose to function properly. That's why severe untreated lows can cause a loss of consciousness. Other symptoms of hypoglycemia include:

- Shakiness (trembling hands, etc.)
- Dizziness or lightheadedness
- Headache
- Hunger
- Heart palpitations
- Sudden sweating
- Clammy or pale skin
- Irritability or unexplained mood swings
- Confusion or disorientation

Treating a Hypo

Once your blood glucose meter has confirmed a low, take action immediately. The rule of thumb for treating a low blood sugar is to take 15 grams of a fast-acting carb, wait fifteen minutes, and test again. Good, quick carb options are three glucose tablets, a half glass of orange juice, or a tube of decorative cake frosting. Candy like Sweet Tarts, Spree, Smarties, and Life Savers are also effective and portable choices. If your levels are still too low after testing the second time, have another 15 grams of carbs. Anytime you don't have your glucose monitor with you to check your blood but feel the symptoms of a hypo, trust your instincts and assume your glucose levels are low.

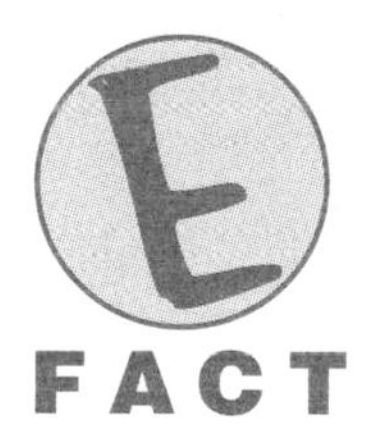

Fat can delay the absorption of sugar, so if you're treating a low, things like donuts, chocolate bars, and ice cream aren't the best choices. While they will do in a pinch, they will take longer to bring glucose back up. Instead, keep a roll of glucose tablets or a tube of glucose gel in your purse, car, and desk, and you'll always be prepared.

It is possible to lose consciousness and/or have a seizure when blood glucose levels drop extremely low. For this reason, it's always a good idea to have someone accessible (e.g., spouse, friend, coworker, teacher) who knows exactly what to do in case of a hypoglycemic episode.

If you are still conscious, they can assist you in taking a fast-acting carb by mouth. This should not be attempted if you are unconscious because of the risk of choking. If you lose consciousness, an injection of the hormone glucagon should be administered; if glucagon is not available, someone should call 911 immediately or transport you to the nearest emergency care facility.

How Glucagon Works

Glucagon stimulates the liver to convert stored glycogen back into glucose. A glucagon kit contains a syringe and a vial of powdered glucagon; the fluid in the prefilled syringe is mixed with the powder immediately before use, drawn into the syringe, and then injected like insulin into a large muscle like the thigh or buttock. Glucagon is available by prescription only; your doctor or CDE (certified diabetes educator) can give you a quick lesson on how and when to use it.

Glucagon will not work to treat a low caused by drinking alcohol. It will also not work if there is an insufficient amount of glycogen available in the liver (such as in cases of malnutrition). Glucagon can cause nausea and possible vomiting, so you should let whoever you instruct in its use know that they should place you on your side if you are given glucagon and are still unconscious.

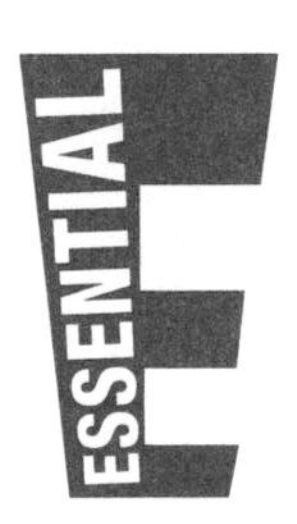

Always store the instructions for your glucagon injection with the syringe. Even with the best preparation, people can forget what they're supposed to be doing in an emotionally charged situation. Make sure you periodically check the expiration date on your glucagon kit, so it is always ready—just in case.

Night Hypos

Even the very idea of having a low in the middle of the night is frightening. Will you wake up? Will your partner wake up? If you have a child with diabetes, how will you know if she has a 2 A.M. hypo? If your blood glucose levels are below 100 mg/dl at bedtime, you may experience a low during the night. Fortunately, with a little planning and treatment adjustments, the problem is usually remedied relatively easily.

Nighttime lows are most common in people taking insulin. You pump out less glucose between midnight and 3 A.M. because your body is at rest and simply doesn't need it. If your insulin peaks during the time when glucose production is unusually low, a hypo could result.

Exercise could again be the culprit if you're working out intensely in the evening. Try a workout earlier in the day, or talk to your doctor about adjusting your insulin dose before working out to accommodate the natural drop in blood sugar that exercise produces.

A bedtime snack can often ward off middle-of-the-night drops in some people. The snack should contain protein to lengthen the release of the carbohydrate. If you are on insulin and nighttime lows persist despite treatment adjustments, an insulin pump (which can be programmed to avoid highs and lows even while you sleep) may be an option.

If you're experiencing night lows, it's a good idea to set your alarm to wake you up for several tests during the middle of the night until you've found a treatment approach that works well for you. Make sure you have glucose tablets or another quick carb on your nightstand just in case you need it. Track the testing info and review it with your doctor to try to find a pattern to your lows.

If you're having elevated morning readings, you may have to do a little detective work and set your alarm for several nighttime tests in order to figure out exactly what's happening. Talk to your doctor about recommendations for adjusting your insulin or treatment.

Sometimes lows that occur when you sleep cause morning fasting blood glucose levels (before breakfast) to be elevated. This phenomenon, known as the *Somogyi effect* or *rebound*, happens when the body starts producing glucagon and epinephrine in response to a low. These hormones signal the liver to convert glycogen to glucose, and the result is high blood sugars upon waking. If your blood glucose is elevated at your first morning test, there's a possibility it's due to an undetected nighttime low. However, it may also be a result of the *dawn phenomenon,* which is a morning high caused by the natural release of blood glucose in the early-morning hours.

Hypoglycemic Unawareness

Sometimes people who have had diabetes for many years develop hypoglycemic unawareness—blood glucose lows that you don't know about because you don't show any symptoms. This may be caused in part by damage to the sympathetic nervous system (called autonomic neuropathy), in which the typical involuntary reactions to low blood sugars—such as sweating and flushing—don't occur. For some people with this condition, a loss of consciousness is their first and only sign that their blood glucose has dipped dangerously low.

Another situation that can trigger hypoglycemic unawareness in some patients is a regimen of intensive or tight blood glucose control. These patients are three times more likely to experience hypoglycemic unawareness than those on a nonintensive treatment program. If you have a hypo, your risk of having yet another low is higher for up to two days following the episode. If you're trying to keep your blood sugars in tight control, you have a fine line to walk, and it's possible to end up in a vicious cycle of low after low. Eventually, hypoglycemic unawareness may result.

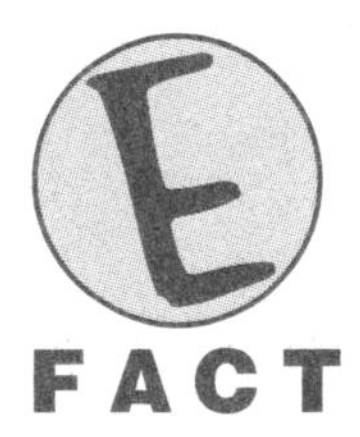

FACT

Several studies have found that moderate intake of caffeine may be useful in heightening sensitivity to symptoms of blood glucose lows in those patients with hypoglycemic unawareness. Be sure to check with your doctor first, as too much caffeine can have negative consequences, particularly if you have high blood pressure.

If you develop hypoglycemic unawareness while on an intensive control program, your doctor will probably recommend increasing your target blood glucose levels slightly to avoid dangerous lows. Some clinical studies have shown that loosening control to allow blood glucose levels to run slightly high for two to three weeks can restore hypoglycemia awareness in some patients. Blood glucose awareness training may also be an option for you if you have hypoglycemic unawareness. Frequent monitoring, increased awareness of hypo triggers, and recognition of some of the subtler signs of a low are the focus of this type of training.

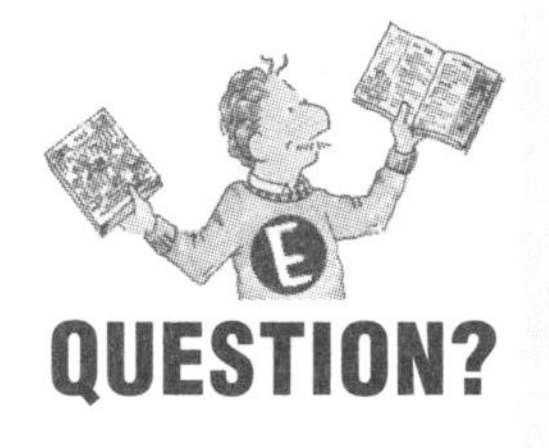

QUESTION?

I've heard that the GlucoWatch can help stop lows at night. Is that true?

The GlucoWatch Biographer (Cygnus), a continuous blood monitoring system that was approved by the FDA in 2001, can detect episodes of hypoglycemia, and several studies have demonstrated that it can reduce the incidence of nighttime hypoglycemic episodes in children. However, you should always follow up any low glucose alarms with a regular finger stick glucose test, as the GlucoWatch can give false positive readings.

Anyone who experiences blood glucose readings of 50 mg/dl or less without any signs of hypoglycemia should let their doctor know promptly.

Diabetic Ketoacidosis (DKA)

On the other end of the spectrum is hyperglycemia, or blood glucose highs. If glucose levels reach 250 mg/dl (13.9 mmol/l) or higher and ketones are present in the blood or urine, these may be indications that diabetic ketoacidosis (DKA) has occurred.

DKA is most common in type 1 diabetes, although it can also occur in people with type 2. It happens when, in the absolute or relative deficiency of insulin (which enables the body to use glucose for energy), the body starts to break down fat for energy instead. Fat metabolism causes ketone bodies to form, throwing the acid balance off kilter in the bloodstream. Meanwhile, the liver continues to pump out more and more glucose in a fruitless attempt to fuel the body, and blood glucose climbs higher and higher. The result is ketoacidosis.

When the body is under a severe degree of stress, hyperglycemia and possible DKA is a danger. Infection, injury, surgical procedures, and even a simple cold or flu are all known offenders in causing blood glucose to rise. Sometimes, people skip their insulin or medication because they are ill, which boosts blood glucose even higher. Dehydration caused by vomiting and diarrhea can also worsen blood glucose levels.

Eating disorders can also be an underlying cause of DKA, particularly in adolescents with type 1 diabetes. One Joslin Diabetes Center study of women with type 1 found that 31 percent intentionally skipped an insulin dose at some point, while 8.8 percent of those did it regularly. Reasons given for intentionally omitting insulin treatment included fear of weight gain and fear of hypoglycemia. The researchers also hypothesized that emotional issues related to living with chronic diabetes could be a cause of insulin omission.

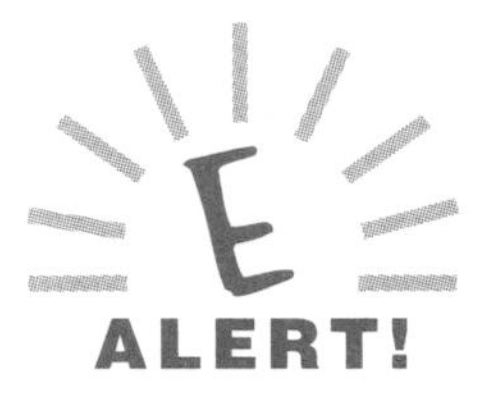

Never skip a dose of insulin or diabetes medication just because you are ill. Illness usually causes blood sugars to climb, and skipping your meds can make the problem worse. In many cases, you may require more insulin when you are ill. Talk to your doctor about a "sick day plan" for your medications and/or insulin dose.

Signs and Symptoms

Often, the symptoms of DKA are ignored initially because many closely resemble the flu or a viral infection. The fact that the flu itself causes blood sugars to rise and can trigger DKA complicates matters further. This is why frequent testing and staying on your treatment schedule is so important when you are ill.

Symptoms of DKA include:

- Fruity smell on the breath (from acetone)
- Nausea
- Vomiting
- Fatigue
- Muscle aches and stiffness
- Abdominal pain
- Extreme thirst and frequent urination
- Rapid breathing or difficulty breathing
- Mental confusion
- Unconsciousness or, in extreme cases, coma

A rare but potentially fatal complication of DKA, cerebral edema (swelling of the brain), is a particular risk in children. Signs of cerebral edema include severe headache, irritability, drowsiness, and confusion.

Treating DKA

Diabetic ketoacidosis should always be treated in a hospital setting. Treatment consists of lowering blood glucose levels with insulin and restoring fluid and electrolyte balance with intravenous saline. In some cases, potassium or other electrolytes may also be administered intravenously. If the underlying cause of the DKA is illness or infection, it should be treated appropriately to prevent recurrence.

When to Test for Ketones

If your blood glucose levels are over 240 mg/dl (13.3 mmol/l), you should test for ketones. Ketone testing is particularly important when you are ill. Home urine tests, which consist of reagent strips that can be dipped in a urine sample and checked against a diagnostic color chart, are easy to perform and are an excellent tool for avoiding DKA. There is also a combination blood glucose and ketone meter (Precision Xtra; MediSense) available in the United States that is useful for home testing. Blood testing for ketones is superior to urine testing, and should be done preferentially.

Hyperglycemic Hyperosmolar Nonketotic Coma (HHNC)

Another complication of extremely high blood glucose levels, hyperosmolar hyperglycemia (also called hyperglycemic hyperosmolar nonketotic coma, or syndrome) occurs most frequently in patients with type 2 diabetes. In HHNC, hyperglycemia occurs without ketosis (the formation of ketone bodies). Extreme dehydration results in a dangerous drop in blood pressure and potential cardiovascular collapse. For this reason, there is a high mortality rate with HHNC.

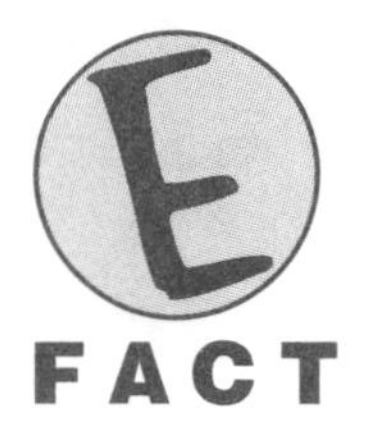

FACT

Certain medications that raise blood glucose levels, such as steroids, atypical antipsychotics, glucocorticoids, and diuretics can cause dangerous hyperglycemic episodes.

Often, people who develop HHNC are on drugs that raise their blood glucose levels, or become dehydrated due to diuretic medications or illness. The condition occurs commonly in elderly patients with previously undiagnosed diabetes. Having impaired kidney function also increases your risk of developing HHNC.

HHNC can occur at blood glucose levels about 600 mg/dl (33.3 mmol/l). At diagnosis, plasma glucose is usually much higher than in DKA (near 1000 mg/dl, or 55.5 mmol/l).

Signs and Symptoms

As opposed to DKA, which usually has a rapid onset, HHNC may be subtler, taking days to weeks to build up to a crisis point. If you are ill and your glucose levels are persistently above 240 mg/dl, even if you test negative for ketones, you should still call your doctor for further advice. If you exhibit any of the signs of HHNC along with elevated blood sugar levels, call your doctor immediately or go to the nearest emergency care facility.

Possible symptoms of HHNC include:

- Frequent urination
- Excessive thirst
- Nausea and vomiting
- Weight loss
- Dehydration
- Weakness
- Seizures
- Confusion, unconsciousness, or coma

Treating HHNC

Treatment for HHNC is similar to that for diabetic ketoacidosis. Restoring the fluid balance to the bloodstream is the immediate goal. A saline solution is administered via an intravenous line, and electrolytes may also be administered. Insulin therapy may or may not be needed. Finding out the root cause or event that precipitated the HHNC is key to preventing its recurrence. HHNC has a significantly higher fatality rate, and must always be treated in the hospital.

High-Risk Situations

There are several situations that cause blood glucose levels to nose-dive or skyrocket. Being prepared for them when and if they occur is the best way to avoid the possible highs and lows.

Sick Days

Being ill is a big risk factor for high blood glucose levels. If your doctor hasn't discussed it with you already, you should ask him about a sick day plan, which is simply a course of action to take if you develop the flu or another mild illness. Here are some guidelines to follow when you are sick:

- **Keep eating and drinking.** Have plenty of nonperishable food and drinks on hand that are easy on the tummy, including Jell-O, broth soups, saltine crackers, fruit juice, and pudding. Drink plenty of water and fluids to avoid dehydration.
- **Stock up the medicine cabinet.** In addition to your glucose meter, you should always have ketone-testing supplies on hand, plus basics like a thermometer and medications to treat diarrhea and vomiting. Talk to your doctor about recommendations for the latter.
- **Stay in touch.** Discuss guidelines with your doctor about when you should call (e.g., if your blood glucose reaches a certain landmark, or if you can't keep food down, or if you exhibit specific symptoms). When in doubt, always pick up the phone.

- **Test often.** Stating the obvious–you'll need to test frequently to pick up dangerous highs early.
- **Don't skip your meds.** Keep taking both insulin and oral medications, and if they aren't bringing down your glucose adequately, call your doctor to discuss increasing the dose.

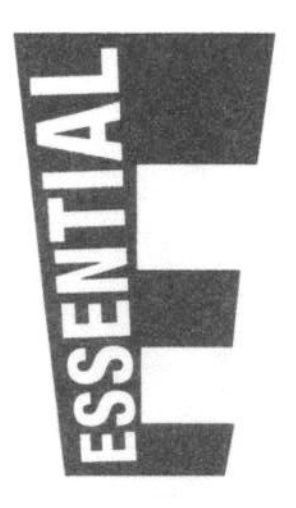

People with diabetes should follow the same alcohol intake guidelines as recommended for the general population—a maximum of one drink daily for women and two drinks a day for men. It takes the body up to two hours to metabolize, or clear, 1 ounce of alcohol from the body, so test frequently after you drink.

Drinking Alcohol

When you drink, your liver shuts down its regular glycogen storage and glucose production operation, opting instead to concentrate on clearing the alcohol from your body. The result can be hypoglycemia, either while you're drinking or hours afterward while your liver continues to clear alcohol from the bloodstream. For this reason, you should always eat when you drink, and be on the lookout for symptoms of a low.

If you choose to drink alcohol, it is absolutely essential that you have a nondrinking friend with you who knows how to recognize the symptoms of hypoglycemia and treat them appropriately. Because alcohol can so easily impair judgment, this should be a person you can trust not to drink.

Always eat something when you drink to keep glucose levels up, and be sure to assess any mixed drinks for "hidden" calories and sugar from fruit juices or mixes (and work them into your overall meal plan). A snack before bed is also important if you've indulged to ward off overnight lows. And when you've been drinking, it's always a good idea to set your alarm to awaken you for a middle of the night blood test for the same reason.

Even if you choose to abstain or have only one drink, but attend a function where the alcohol is flowing freely, it's important to have a designated (non)drinking buddy who knows what to look out for. Some of the symptoms of a low–confusion, mood swings, and incoherence–can easily be mistaken for intoxication by others (especially if they've had a few themselves) and not treated appropriately.

Medications

Certain medications can cause highs or lows. Whenever you get a new prescription, ask your doctor about its potential to impact your blood glucose levels and what adjustments you can make to your treatment to avoid a blood sugar emergency. And for the same reason, never take supplements or herbal remedies without running them by your doctor first.

Make sure you are never caught without your diabetes medication. Always get your insulin and oral drug prescriptions filled well before you run out. If you ever find yourself in the position of not being able to afford your medication, call your doctor and explain your circumstances. In many cases, she may be able to offer you drug samples to get you through a particularly difficult time. She may also be able to prescribe a less-expensive generic or alternative drug.

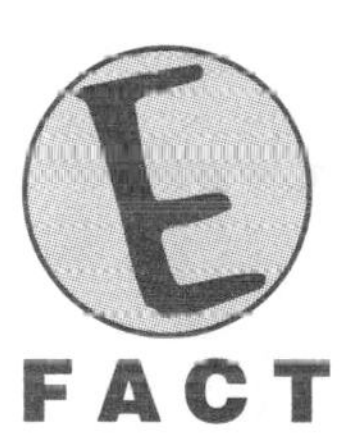

FACT

There are several patient assistance programs available through major pharmaceutical manufacturers that offer drugs to those who need them at a reduced rate or free of charge. Ask your doctor or see Appendix A for more information.

Buddy System

Embarrassed, ashamed, self-conscious, guilty, alone—do any of these describe the way you're feeling about having diabetes? First of all, realize that you aren't to blame for having this disease. These feelings are a natural part of coming to terms with your diagnosis. It may take some time to overcome them completely, but in the meantime you need to get past them enough to let the people around you know you need their help.

As of the writing of this book, there were 17 million people living with diabetes in America. That makes the odds pretty darn good that at least a few of your coworkers, neighbors, friends, and family have already been touched by the disease on some level. With that in mind, you may not need to tell them a lot they don't already know; then again, they may be sorely in need of some accurate and current diabetes education. Either way, you only have to share the basics of handling an emergency at this point.

First off, have a "buddy" (or two or three) at each place you frequent regularly, such as work, the gym or playing field, class, church, etc. Let them know (and give them access to) where you keep your basic supplies (i.e., meter, fast-acting glucose, glucagon kit) and provide them with instructions on administering glucagon. Most of the glucagon kits on the market have illustrated instructions with them that make giving an injection easier.

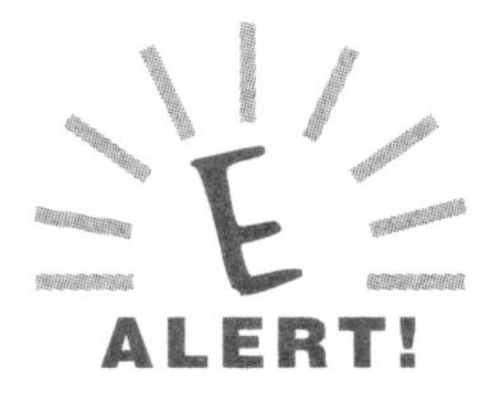

When educating friends, family, and coworkers about emergency situations, make sure they understand the difference between insulin and glucagon. Since both are injected, they may easily be confused, a situation that could have life-threatening consequences if you were to lose consciousness and were treated with the wrong drug.

These basic guidelines can give them direction for offering you assistance. Customize them to your own particular blood sugar numbers:

- If I look ill or am acting strange, ask me if I'm okay and suggest that I check my blood sugars.
- If I test low (under 70 mg/dl or as indicated by a low alarm on my meter) and am still conscious, help me to eat or drink some glucose tablets, juice, or other fast-acting sugars.
- If I test extremely high (over 240 mg/dl or as indicated by a high alarm on my meter) and I lose consciousness or am incoherent, call 911 or get me to an emergency room immediately.
- If I test low and lose consciousness, do not try to feed me. Call 911 immediately and administer a glucagon injection.
- If I haven't tested or you don't know what my blood sugar levels were and I lose consciousness, never try to feed me or give me insulin or glucagon. Instead, call 911 immediately.

Medical Identification

Even if you've got a buddy with you at all times, it's important to make sure that you have medical identification in case you need to be treated by medical personnel. You don't need to sport a giant scarlet *D* on your lapel, but wearing some form of ID at all times is the best way to ensure you will get proper treatment should a blood sugar emergency cause you to lose consciousness among strangers.

It may be tempting to take off your ID at the gym or before a run. Don't. During (and following) exercise is a high-risk time for hypoglycemia. The same goes for social events and parties with alcohol. Living with diabetes means that blood sugar lows and highs can strike any time. Don't be caught unprepared.

The Options

When you're shopping for a medical ID, keep these elements in mind:

- It must be noticeable—the most important criterion for a good ID.
- It must be comfortable—otherwise you won't wear it.
- It should be durable enough to stand up to sun, surf, and whatever other elements you may encounter.
- It should be comprehensive—make sure it lists all pertinent medical information.
- It should be stylish. Make sure you like it, or, again, you won't wear it.

Your ID should indicate that you have diabetes. If you take insulin, it should say that as well, along with any drug allergies you may have. Your tag will let paramedics and other health care providers know that they should test your blood glucose before treating you.

What Works and What Doesn't

Some people don't like to shout out "I have diabetes!" and opt for less intrusive means of identification like a key chain or a wallet card. Unfortunately, being subtle doesn't do you a whole lot of good in an emergency situation. If you collapse, probably the only person that would go immediately for your wallet or your car keys would be a mugger or carjacker. A medical alert bracelet, pendant, or watchband is much more likely to get noticed for the right reason.

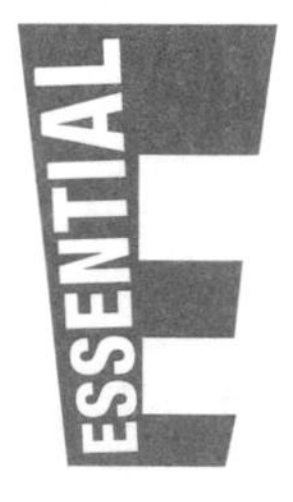

Make it a habit to always test your blood glucose before you drive. If it's too low, treat it and wait for the subsequent rise before turning on the ignition. Even the slightest lapse in concentration can have serious repercussions behind the wheel of a car. Driving with a blood glucose low can be just as dangerous as drinking and driving.

Most medical IDs are marked with a caduceus, a winged staff entwined with snakes that is the Greek symbol for medicine. Today's medical ID products are available in a wide variety of configurations, including watch tags, bracelets, pendants, sports bands, shoelace tags, clip-on ID cards, custom-made gemstone jewelry, and even temporary tattoos. Products like shoelace tags (which are worn securely at the toe end of the laces) are good choices for young children who may not like to wear bracelets or pendants.

Emergency Response Services

If you have a complicated medical history, or simply want to have more peace of mind regarding treatment of your diabetes in an emergency, you can invest in a subscription to an emergency response service like Medic-Alert. These companies store your detailed medical information in a database, then issue you medical identification engraved with both your medical condition and their toll-free number. When hospital or emergency personnel call the number, your information can be relayed to them. If you aren't willing or able to make an investment in this type of service, some standard ID products feature compartments for storing more extensive written medical information.

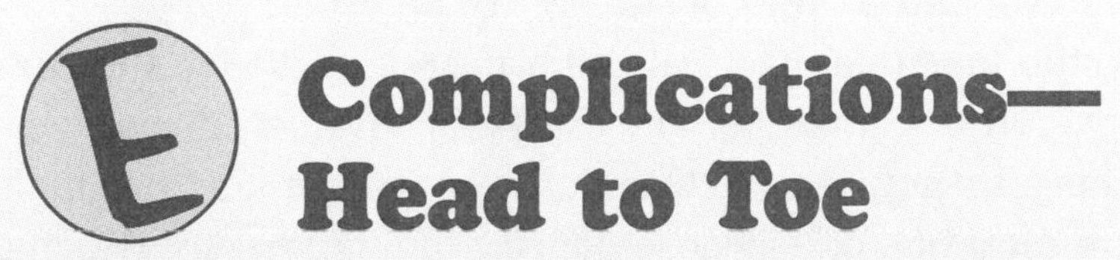

Chapter 15

Complications—Head to Toe

Your body is equipped with 60,000 miles of blood vessels and wired with a whopping 100,000 miles of nerve fibers. A clog here, some corrosion there, and all this hardware suffers from the strain. Diabetes is like a bad tenant, backing up pipes and short-circuiting wiring. You may not be able to evict it, but you can do your part to prevent long-term systemic complications with proper maintenance.

Neurological Complications

Diabetes is a risk factor for stroke, nerve damage, and cognitive impairment. While stroke is technically a cardiovascular complication caused by a blockage of blood to or a hemorrhage in the brain, it can cause impairment to memory, vision, speech, movement, and other brain functions in varying degrees of severity.

The other major neurological complications of diabetes are caused by neuropathy, or nerve damage. The exact way in which diabetes causes nerve damage is not completely understood yet, but it's thought that over time, high levels of blood glucose damage the nerve cells, which unlike other cells don't require an insulin "key" to allow glucose inside them. Researchers have also hypothesized that too much glucose causes depletion of nitric acid, which in turn cuts off blood supply to the nerves.

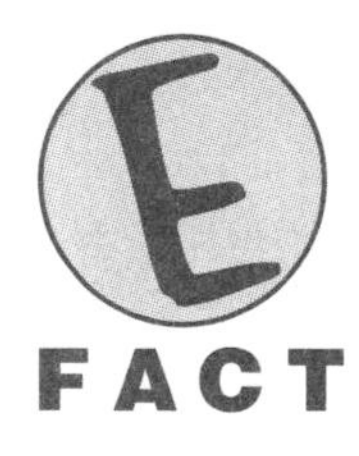

FACT

Neuropathies are either *diffuse* (affecting a wide area or several areas of the body) or *focal* (affecting a specific place on the body). Most neuropathic conditions related to diabetes are diffuse, including peripheral and autonomic neuropathy.

Peripheral Neuropathy (PN)

Peripheral neuropathy is often called stocking-glove syndrome because it most commonly affects the feet and hands. The condition can be particularly troublesome in the feet because of the chance that you may develop an injury that you don't notice, and compound the problem through the simple act of walking (for more on PN and your feet, see Chapter 16).

Symptoms of peripheral neuropathy include:

- A feeling of "pins and needles"
- Tingling and/or burning sensations
- In some people, pain
- Numbness
- Balance problems (if PN is present in the feet)
- Reflex problems and muscle weakness

Antidepressant medications (amitriptyline and desipramine) may be useful in blocking pain signals, although side effects may be an issue for some patients. Neurontin (gabapentin, an anticonvulsant) is an effective treatment for many people with PN and has the additional advantage of having few side effects. A number of studies have also shown promising treatment results with alpha lipoic acid (ALA) treatment, although ALA is not FDA approved for this particular "off-label" use at this point in time.

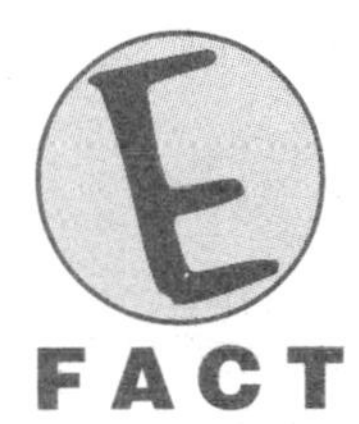
FACT

Over half of men with diabetes over age fifty have impotence problems, which can be related to both neuropathy and cardiovascular complications. In women, diabetes can impact estrogen levels, menstrual and ovulation cycles, and sexual desire.

Treatment with lidocaine or with capsaicin cream, which contains a substance derived from hot peppers that helps to block pain signals, may also be recommended by your doctor. And some anecdotal success has been reported in treating PN with acupuncture and with transcutaneous electronic nerve stimulations (TENS), which uses electricity to block pain signals.

Autonomic Neuropathy

While many people with diabetes are aware of the signs and symptoms of PN, significantly fewer are educated about, or tested for, autonomic neuropathy. A stealth disorder, autonomic neuropathy short-circuits the nerves that control the sympathetic (autonomic, or involuntary) nervous system. Blood pressure, heart rate, perspiration, salivation, gastrointestinal and bladder function, sexual potency, and vision can all be impaired by autonomic neuropathy damage.

Autonomic neuropathy causes a wide spectrum of nonspecific symptoms ranging from constipation and diarrhea to dizziness and excessive perspiration (see Autonomic Neuropathy table). Unfortunately, these are also common signs of a number of medical conditions, which makes autonomic neuropathy particularly difficult to detect without regular screening. Often, a diagnosis isn't made until organ damage has occurred.

Autonomic Neuropathy		
	Symptoms	**Possible Associated Complications**
Cardiovascular system	Dizziness Drop in blood pressure Less variation than normal in heart rate Elevated resting heart rate Shortness of breath Perspiration	Orthostatic hypotension Silent heart attack Serious heart rhythm abnormalities
Digestive system	Constipation Diarrhea Bloating and nausea Premature feeling of fullness	Gastroparesis
Genitourinary	Urinary tract infections Urinary incontinence Vaginal dryness Inability to maintain erection Decreased or increased urination	Neurogenic bladder Impotence
Sudomotor system	Increased perspiration (trunk and face) Decreased perspiration (extremities) Dry, thick skin on hands and feet	Skin rashes and infection
Vision	Small pupils No pupil response to light/dark	Impaired night vision

Cardiovascular Autonomic Neuropathy (CAN)

This disorder begins silently without symptoms of chest pain or discomfort (angina), and often remains undetected until serious myocardial infarction (death of the heart muscle due to lack of oxygen) has occurred. As a result, these "silent heart attacks" often pass without proper medical attention.

If you experience any unexplained shortness of breath, weakness and fatigue, and/or excessive perspiration—all possible symptoms of silent heart attack—report it to your doctor promptly. The mortality rate of CAN is up to 50 percent within five years once symptoms appear, so early diagnosis is essential.

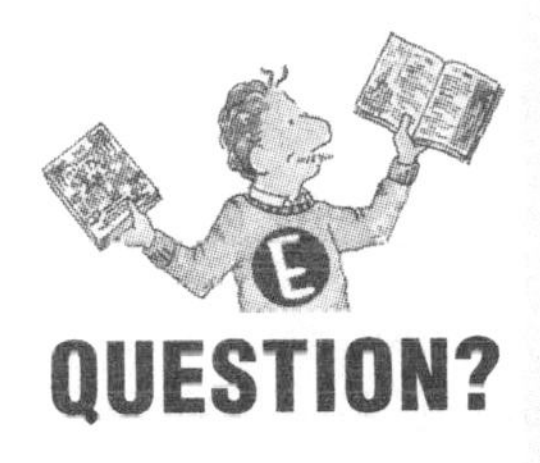

QUESTION?

I get dizzy when I stand suddenly, and my doc said it could be neuropathy. Isn't that a foot condition?

Your doctor is talking about autonomic neuropathy. Cardiovascular autonomic neuropathy can trigger a sudden drop in blood pressure known as orthostatic (postural) hypotension. When you stand up, blood vessel and nerve damage prevent your blood pressure from rising quickly enough to compensate for the change in position, and dizziness, vision problems, and lightheadedness result.

Patients with CAN have little variation in their heart rate, which typically remains continuously elevated both at rest and under stress (e.g., after exercise). Heart rate variability (HRV) testing is used to diagnose the condition. HRV testing involves assessing the heart rate with an electrocardiograph during activities of deep breathing, a postural test (i.e., lying down, rising, and standing), and the Valsalva maneuver. The Valsalva maneuver is performed by bearing down, or forcefully breathing out through the mouth with both the mouth and nose closed. In patients without CAN, the heart rate should slow during this maneuver. If heart rate remains consistent (i.e., does not slow or speed up) during all three of these activities, CAN is suspected.

Autonomic neuropathy can also cause hypoglycemic unawareness, a potentially serious inability to detect the physical symptoms of a low blood glucose episode.

Cognitive Impairment

People with diabetes may experience memory problems and cognitive impairment, but it isn't completely clear whether these problems are a result of physical processes, the social and psychological toll of the disease, or a combination of the two.

There is some evidence that impaired glucose tolerance, a precursor to type 2 diabetes, can cause memory loss and atrophy of the hippocampus (the part of the brain responsible for learning and memory). Research has also indicated a greater risk for cognitive impairment in people with type 1 diabetes, possibly because of their increased risk for and incidence of hypoglycemia.

There are plenty of medical reasons for children and their parents to avoid hypoglycemia, of course, but researchers disagree on whether long-term cognitive dysfunction is one of them. Some studies have shown a connection between severe hypoglycemia and learning difficulties in children with type 1 diabetes, but others have contradicted this finding.

Musculoskeletal Complications

In addition to peripheral neuropathy, there are several other complications of diabetes that affect the musculoskeletal system and the extremities.

Frozen Shoulder

Frozen shoulder, or adhesive capsulitis, is a disorder of the connective tissue that limits the normal range of motion of the shoulder. In diabetes, it is caused by changes to the collagen in the shoulder joint as a result of long-term hyperglycemia. It usually happens in one shoulder only, although it can occur in both.

Physical therapy focused on improving range of motion, along with anti-inflammatory medications, are usually the first line of treatment for frozen shoulder. Cortisone injections are also sometimes used in treating frozen shoulder.

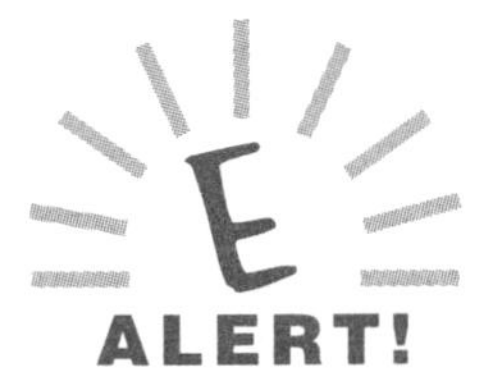

Conditions involving inflammation of the tendons or joints are sometimes treated with nonsteroidal anti-inflammatory medications (NSAIDs) like ibuprofen or naproxen. However, NSAIDs should be prescribed with care in patients with kidney disease and/or cardiovascular disease, as they have the potential to worsen these conditions.

Dupuytren's Contracture

Another condition that limits range of motion is Dupuytren's contracture. As its common name—trigger finger—suggests, the condition is characterized by pain, stiffness, and a "locking" of the index finger. The tendon in the finger becomes inflamed and the tendon sheath, or covering, is damaged. Flexing the finger becomes increasingly difficult, and eventually the finger may lock up in a "trigger pull" position. Again, anti-inflammatories and physical therapy may be prescribed. In some cases, surgery may be required to correct the condition.

Carpal Tunnel Syndrome

Often confused with or mistaken for peripheral neuropathy, carpal tunnel syndrome involves nerve entrapment rather than nerve damage. The medial nerve (a nerve that runs through your wrist) becomes compressed, or entrapped, in the ligaments that surround it (the carpal tunnel). This can be caused by repetitive stress (such as that caused by typing at a keyboard or playing guitar), and is exacerbated by diabetes because high blood glucose can cause changes to the collagen in the ligaments, making entrapment more likely.

The result is tingling, "pins and needles," and burning sensations similar to what you might feel in PN. In fact, your doctor may refer to it as a *compression neuropathy* because it causes these symptoms. The difference is that carpal tunnel usually affects just the first three fingers of the hand (thumb, index, and middle fingers; although sometimes the half of the ring finger closest to the middle finger is involved), while PN involves the entire hand.

Carpal tunnel syndrome is treated with wrist splints and sometimes corticosteroid injections. In some cases, surgery may be required to relieve pressure on the medial nerve.

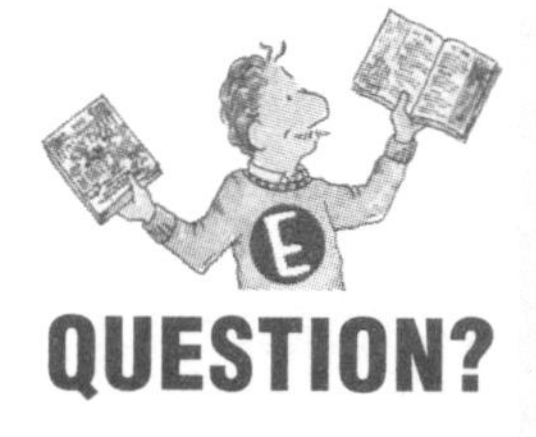

QUESTION?

What is stiff-hand syndrome, and how can I treat it?
Stiff-hand syndrome (digital sclerosis) is caused by a buildup of collagen under the skin. It generally doesn't cause any pain, but it can affect your flexibility. Talk to your doctor or physical therapist about a regimen of hand-stretching exercises that may help relieve the stiffness. Paraffin wax is also used as a treatment sometimes, but should only be applied by a health care professional because of the risk of burns.

Cardiovascular Complications

According to the U.S. Centers for Disease Control (CDC), a staggering 65 percent of people with diabetes die from heart disease or stroke, yet few people with diabetes are aware of their increased cardiovascular risks.

Bringing blood glucose, blood pressure, and LDL cholesterol levels down is the best way to combat diabetes-related cardiovascular complications. The National Diabetes Education Program (NDEP) and the Department of Health and Human Services (HHS) recommend following the "ABCs" of diabetes treatment to maintain optimal heart health.

ABCs of Diabetes Treatment		
A	A1c	<7 percent
B	Blood pressure	<130/80 mmHg
C	Cholesterol	LDL <100 mg/dl

For patients with a poor cholesterol profile, dietary adjustments (i.e., lowering intake of saturated fat) and increased exercise are recommended. If these don't provide sufficient improvement, or if LDL and/or triglyceride levels are significantly elevated to begin with, drugs called statins—such as Lipitor (atorvastatin), Pravachol (pravastatin), or Zocor (simvastatin)—may be prescribed.

Atherosclerosis and CAD

Atherosclerosis, more commonly known as hardening or clogging of the arteries, is caused by a buildup of fatty material (also called plaque or cholesterol), which restricts blood flow. For patients with arterial obstructions, medications such as nitroglycerin, beta-blockers, and angiotensin-converting enzyme (ACE) inhibitors may be prescribed.

Blockage to the arteries that feed the heart is called coronary artery disease (CAD). What makes CAD particularly dangerous is that symptoms don't typically appear until vessels are significantly blocked. Symptoms of CAD include:

- Chest pain (angina)
- Pain in the left arm or shoulder (referred pain)
- Neck or jaw pain
- Chest tightness or pressure
- Shortness of breath
- Nausea
- Perspiration
- Irregular heartbeat (arrhythmia)

An electrocardiogram (ECG), echocardiogram, and/or stress test may be helpful in diagnosing blocked arteries. If CAD is left untreated, the artery may become completely blocked. When blood flow is severely restricted to the heart, or completely blocked off, myocardial infarction (heart attack) occurs. Without oxygen from the blood, the affected area of heart muscle dies. Symptoms of a heart attack are the same as those described previously for CAD, except the pain is considerably more intense, and the symptoms prolonged. However, in people with diabetes who suffer from autonomic neuropathy, pain symptoms may not be felt at all, resulting in a "silent heart attack."

In cases of stroke or heart attack, where restoring blood flow is critical to prevent tissue death and damage, clot-dissolving or "clot-busting" (fibrinolytic or thrombolytic) drugs may be administered–such as Activase (alteplase), Streptase (streptokinase), Abbokinase (urokinase), Eminase (anistreplase), or Retavase (reteplase).

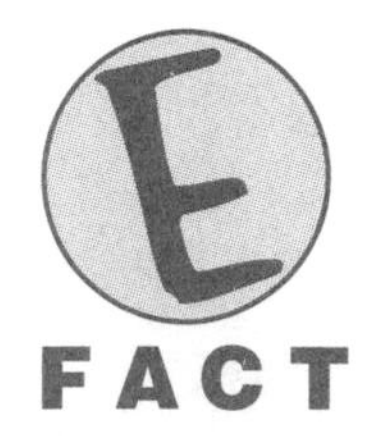
FACT

In those at risk, an aspirin a day may keep heart disease away. The ADA recommends that adult men and women with a history of or risk factors for CAD, PVD, stroke, or heart attack take a daily dose of 81 to 325 milligrams of coated aspirin. Aspirin therapy is not recommended for those with aspirin allergy, liver problems, bleeding disorders, or young people.

You may also require an angioplasty, a procedure in which a catheter is inserted into the artery and an attached balloon is expanded to clear the blockage. Sometimes, a device called a stent, which is expanded inside the artery to hold the vessel open, is used. Atherectomy, a procedure that strips fatty blockages out of the artery, may also be performed.

Studies have indicated that coronary bypass surgery may have better long-term outcomes than angioplasty for people with diabetes. Bypass involves rerouting the circulation by grafting a healthy piece of artery onto the obstructed blood vessel and around the blockage.

Peripheral Vascular Disease (PVD)

Like CAD, peripheral vascular disease (also called peripheral arterial disease, or PAD) involves atherosclerosis. Unlike CAD, PVD affects the extremities–most commonly the legs. Signs of PVD include:

- Calf and leg cramps, usually when walking (intermittent claudication)
- Smooth, shiny, hairless skin on the shins
- Chronically cold feet and legs
- Numb legs or feet
- A bluish or reddish cast to the skin of the feet and/or legs
- Sores or ulcers on the legs that won't heal

The treatment of PVD is similar to that of CAD. Weight loss, cholesterol improvement through diet or drug therapy, appropriate exercise, and medication may all be recommended. Good foot care, important for everyone with diabetes, is especially essential to those people who develop PVD.

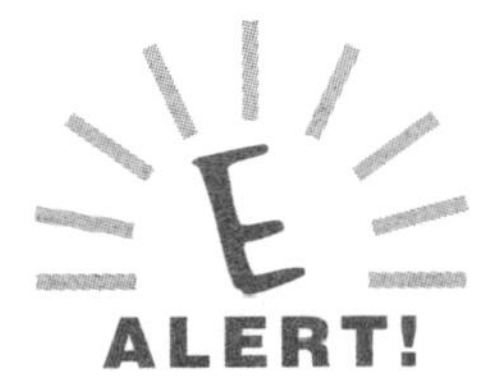

Congestive heart failure (CHF) is yet another cardiovascular condition that people with diabetes are at a higher risk for. Symptoms include fluid retention (edema), shortness of breath, heart palpitations, fatigue, and low tolerance for exercise. CHF is usually treated with ACE inhibitors, digoxin, and diuretics. In some cases, beta-blockers may also be prescribed.

Hypertension

Another leading complication on the diabetes hit parade is hypertension, or high blood pressure. It occurs in up to 65 percent of people with diabetes, and is also closely linked with both diabetic kidney disease and CAD, making it a complex yet critical-to-manage condition.

The ADA recommends that nonpregnant adults with diabetes age eighteen years and older aim for a blood pressure goal of less than 130 mmHg systolic and less than 80 mmHg diastolic (commonly expressed as 130/80 or "130 over 80"). A patient is considered hypertensive if he or she has a blood pressure reading greater than or equal to 140/90 mmHg. Weight loss, smoking cessation, exercise, and dietary adjustments such as lowering sodium may all be part of your recommended treatment program if your blood pressure is elevated. Since these are largely all goals of your diabetes management program to begin with, it may make them easier to accomplish.

If lifestyle modifications don't bring down your blood pressure, medications such as angiotensin-converting enzyme (ACE) inhibitors, beta-blockers, diuretics, and angiotensin receptor blockers (ARBs) are effective options for some people. ACE inhibitors have also been shown to have the added benefit of delaying the progression of kidney disease, and may be a preferred therapy in patients who also have renal impairment. Your doctor can tell you more about these drugs and if they may be right for you.

Stroke

Another potential cardiovascular complication of diabetes is ischemic stroke. Ischemic stroke occurs when an artery leading to the brain becomes blocked and blood flow is cut off. Symptoms of stroke hit suddenly and include the following:

- Weakness or numbness of the arm, face, or leg (usually one-sided)
- Mental confusion
- Difficulty speaking
- Dizziness and/or problems with balance
- Visual problems
- Severe headache

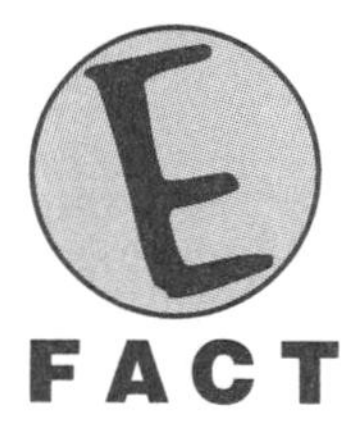

FACT

If you have diabetes, you are at higher risk for a transient ischemic attack (TIA, or ministroke). A TIA is characterized by the typical symptoms of stroke, but it resolves on its own without treatment. If you think you've had a TIA, tell your doctor immediately. It is a warning sign that something is wrong, and you are at risk for a full-blown stroke.

Because of the complex relationships between diabetes and all the systems of the body, many diabetic complications are interrelated. For example, University of Wisconsin research (the Atherosclerosis Risk in Communities Study) found that middle-aged people who had never experienced a stroke but suffered from retinopathy displayed poorer cognitive function that those who didn't have retinopathy. The finding suggests that cerebral microvascular disease (which is at the root of diabetic retinopathy) may contribute to the development of cognitive impairment, even when stroke doesn't occur.

Visual Complications

The longer you have had diabetes, the greater your risk for visual complications from the disease. Nearly everyone who has type 1 diabetes, and the majority of those with type 2 diabetes, will experience some degree of retinopathy in their lifetime. The good news is that early diagnosis and treatment with laser surgery can prevent serious vision loss in the majority of cases.

Retinopathy

According to the ADA, diabetic retinopathy is the primary cause of new-onset blindness for adults between ages twenty and seventy-four. The condition is caused by blockage and/or leaking of the blood vessels that feed the retina of the eye. Swelling of the macula, part of the retina, is called macular edema, and is a possible complication that can cause blurred vision. Often, symptoms of retinopathy are not noticed until they reach an advanced, or proliferative, stage.

Laser treatment is usually recommended for treating diabetic retinopathy. Depending on the progression of the disease, lasers may be used to either seal leaky blood vessels or destroy abnormal vessels completely.

A vitrectomy, a surgical procedure that replaces the vitreous fluid of the eye with a clear saline solution, may also be performed if blood vessels have hemorrhaged significantly into the vitreous. Both laser treatment and vitrectomy are outpatient procedures that are performed by an ophthalmologist or eye surgeon.

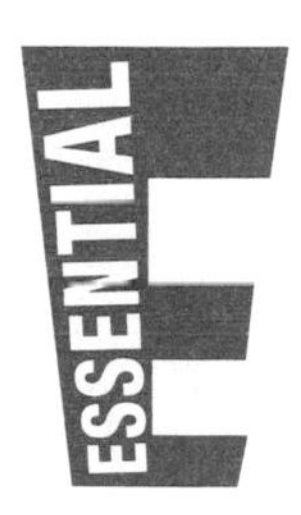

You need a dilated-eye exam at least annually to detect diabetic eye disease early. Other essentials for good eye health include kicking the smoking habit, lowering blood pressure, and keeping your A1c down. The Diabetes Control and Complications Trial (DCCT) found that people with uncontrolled blood glucose levels developed retinopathy four times more frequently than those who practiced tight blood glucose control.

Glaucoma

Glaucoma is caused by pressure buildup in the eye that can damage the optic nerve. In cases where the normal drainage patterns of the eye are blocked, the aqueous fluids of the eye build up and put pressure on the optic nerve. A loss of peripheral (side) vision is often the first sign of glaucoma. Depending on the type of glaucoma, you may also experience severe headache. The condition may be treated with special eye drops that lower the pressure level in the eyes. Laser surgery may also be recommended.

Cataracts

People with diabetes are more likely to develop cataracts at an earlier age than the general population. If you have diabetes, you are also twice as likely to develop the condition. Cataracts are characterized by a clouding of the lens of the eye. Symptoms include cloudy or fuzzy vision, double vision, and sensitivity to bright light.

Mild cataracts may not require surgical intervention, unless vision is significantly reduced. Surgical treatment involves removing the clouded, natural lens and replacing it with a plastic lens that has been calibrated for your vision needs. The prognosis is excellent for anyone undergoing cataract surgery, and the procedure improves vision in an estimated 95 percent of cases. However, there are some risks for people who also have diabetic retinopathy, as lens replacement can cause a worsening of that condition. Your doctor can provide you with information on the risks and benefits of cataract surgery in your specific medical situation.

Kidney Disease

Your kidneys are two of the hardest-working organs in your body, filtering approximately 50 gallons of fluid from the blood that passes through them daily. After the million or so nephrons in each kidney balance electrolytes and filter toxins, 49.5 gallons of fluid are returned to the bloodstream cleansed and chemically and hormonally balanced. The remaining half-gallon leaves the body as urine.

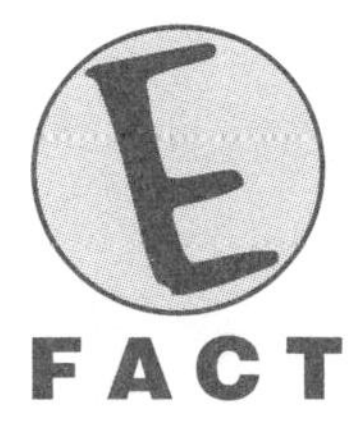

FACT

People of certain ethnic and racial backgrounds are at a higher risk for developing kidney disease, including African-Americans, Hispanics, Mexican-Americans, and Native Americans.

Blood vessel damage and hypertension associated with diabetes can take a serious toll on renal (or kidney) function, damaging this amazing filtration capacity of the kidneys. As a result, diabetes has become the number one cause of end-stage renal disease (ESRD, or chronic kidney failure), accounting for 35 percent of all cases.

Both type 1 and type 2 patients are at risk for developing kidney problems, and the risk of developing ESRD increases with the length of time since diabetes diagnosis, possibly due to the prevalence of high blood pressure in diabetes and the added stress it places on the kidneys. In fact, uncontrolled hypertension is the second most common cause of kidney failure in America, accounting for about 23 percent of the ESRD patient population according to the National Kidney Foundation.

Signs and symptoms of kidney disease include the following:

- Blood and/or protein (albumin) in the urine
- High blood pressure
- Frequent urination, especially at night
- Leg cramps
- Puffiness and swelling around the eyes, hands, and feet (edema)
- Excessive itching (pruritis)
- Nausea and vomiting
- Weakness

If your doctor suspects renal impairment, she will run several diagnostic tests to assess your kidney function, including a urine test for microalbumin, or trace amounts of protein in the urine. Microalbuminuria is one of the hallmarks of early kidney disease, and at one time was thought to be the beginning of the end of kidney function for people with diabetes. However, a Joslin Diabetes Center study published in the *New England Journal of Medicine* in June 2003 found that 58 percent of type

1 study subjects who developed microalbuminuria were actually able to reverse the condition within six years with good control of blood glucose, blood pressure, and cholesterol levels.

Importance of Good Control

Several large-scale diabetes studies have demonstrated that tight blood glucose control can significantly reduce the risk of nephropathy. In fact, the DCCT found that people with type 1 diabetes who maintained an average A1c of 7.2 percent cut their risk of developing nephropathy and other complications up to 75 percent. And the United Kingdom Prospective Diabetes Study (UKPDS) found that people with type 2 diabetes achieved a 35 percent reduction in risk for nephropathy for each percentage point they lowered their A1c levels.

If you develop kidney disease, you may have to watch your protein intake; a registered dietitian can help you to develop a meal plan that is low in dietary protein and compatible with blood sugar control goals. However, studies are still inconclusive on the benefits of low-protein diets in lowering the risk of developing kidney disease, and the ADA currently recommends that most adults who have diabetes *without* known kidney damage include the recommended daily allowance (RDA) of approximately 10 percent of total calories from protein in their diets.

Because diabetic kidney disease often goes hand in hand with hypertension, you may be prescribed ACE inhibitors or other medication to control your blood pressure and cut the workload of your kidneys, as well.

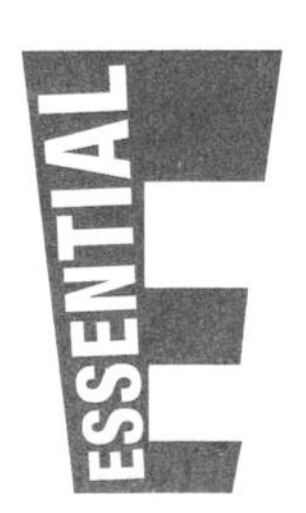

Kidney failure is an irreversible condition. Once kidney function diminishes to less than 10 to 15 percent and ESRD occurs, hemodialysis, peritoneal dialysis, or kidney transplant are the only treatment options.

Digestive Complications

Gastroparesis, or delayed stomach emptying, literally means partial stomach paralysis. It is another type of autonomic neuropathy caused by damage to the vagus nerve, which is responsible for facilitating the passage of food through the digestive system. What makes gastroparesis a particular problem in people with diabetes is that it can greatly hinder your efforts at blood glucose control. If you can't predict how quickly your food will be digested, your insulin or medication could work too quickly or too slowly.

Symptoms of gastroparesis may include:

- Nausea
- Vomiting
- Abdominal bloating
- Weight loss
- Premature feeling of fullness

Dealing with Gastroparesis

People with gastroparesis who take insulin frequently need to adjust their dosage. Insulin lispro (Humalog) may be recommended since it starts working within minutes and peaks within an hour or two. If you have gastroparesis, your doctor can provide specific recommendations for insulin therapy for your particular situation.

Adjustments to diet are also usually necessary to ease gastroparesis. High-fat and high-fiber foods are discouraged since they slow digestion. Your doctor may recommend smaller, more frequent meals, or replacing some meals with liquid-based nutrition. In cases where vomiting is so extreme that you are having trouble keeping food down altogether, parenteral or jejunostomy (tube) feeding may be required.

Jejunostomy involves insertion of a feeding tube through the abdomen and into the small intestine. A liquid nutritional compound is then administered through the tube. Parenteral nutrition uses an intravenous line directly into the bloodstream to provide vital nutrients. It is usually only used as a temporary measure while treatment by other means is stabilized.

For cases that are nonresponsive to dietary changes, injections of botulinum toxin (botox) into the sphincter of the pylorus (the opening connecting the stomach to the small intestine) may be attempted in an effort to relax the opening to let food pass through more readily.

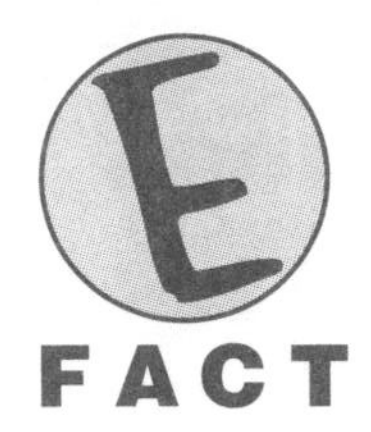

FACT

Gastroparesis occurs most frequently in people with type 1 diabetes, affecting an estimated 20 percent of people with the disease. But it can also occur in type 2 diabetes.

Medication may also be prescribed to try to speed up digestion. Commonly prescribed gastroparesis medications include metoclopramide (Reglan, a muscle stimulant), erythromycin (an antibiotic that can speed stomach emptying), and domperidone (Motilium). Domperidone was not approved for use in the United States as of early 2003, but is available in Canada and Europe. Another medication, cisapride (Propulsid), was withdrawn from the U.S. market by manufacturer Janssen Pharmaceutica in 2000, but is still available for qualified patients through a compassionate use program developed by Janssen and the FDA.

Enterra Therapy (Medtronic), a device that uses electrical impulses to stimulate digestion by the stomach, has been successful in treating chronic gastroparesis in some patients for whom drug therapy was not effective. Often described as a pacemaker for the stomach, Enterra is approved as a Humanitarian Use Device by the FDA as of early 2003. HUD status means that the device is conditionally cleared for use in specific rare diseases and conditions by the FDA.

Skin Problems

There are a number of different skin conditions that can affect people with diabetes. Nerve and small blood vessel damage can make dry skin worse in people with diabetes. Keeping the skin well hydrated is important because any cracks or fissures could easily become infected. In addition to being uncomfortable, the itchiness of dry skin may cause a scratch or abrasion that also poses an infection risk.

Use a humidifier in the home and office, and avoid exposure to harsh detergents and household cleaners that are notorious for drying out skin. If you keep a bottle of hand lotion next to the soap at the kitchen and bathroom sinks, you'll be more likely to remember to use it after each hand washing. Make sure the soap you use for washing is mild.

"Tougher" areas of the skin, such as the soles of the feet, may benefit from a moisturizing lotion containing urea (for moisture) and alpha-hydroxy, or AHA (for sloughing off dead skin). It's a good idea to run any new products past your doctor or CDE first. Certain areas of your body should also be kept dry. Using baby powder in the armpits, between the toes, and other moisture-prone skin fold areas can help to prevent fungal infections.

People with diabetes frequently develop thickened, shiny areas of skin that are caused by changes to the collagen fibers. A tendency toward yellow-tinted skin and nails, too, may be triggered by collagen changes (although the cause of this phenomenon isn't completely understood).

Other skin conditions that are common in people with diabetes include the following:

- **Acanthosis nigricans:** Dark, thickened brown patches in the folds of the skin that are common in overweight people with insulin resistance and type 2 diabetes.
- **Bacterial infections:** Staph or strep infections in the skin that may appear as sties, boils, or cellulitis.
- **Fungal infections:** Usually occur in warm, moist areas such as skin folds. Candidiasis (yeast infection), tinea pedis (athlete's foot or ringworm), and tinea cruris (jock itch or ringworm) are all common fungal infections.
- **Diabetic dermopathy:** Brown, scaly, rounded patches on the skin that frequently appear on the shins and usually heal on their own.
- **Necrobiosis lipoidica diabeticorum:** Changes in the collagen of the skin that cause large, raised, red, shiny, and sometimes itchy spots. If the spots rupture, they will require proper wound care.

Several other, less common, conditions that may occur in the presence of uncontrolled high blood sugars include bullosis diabeticorum (diabetic blisters) and eruptive xanthomatosis (small, yellow, red-ringed bumps), most commonly due to high lipids. Both of these conditions usually resolve themselves once blood glucose levels are brought back under control. (E)

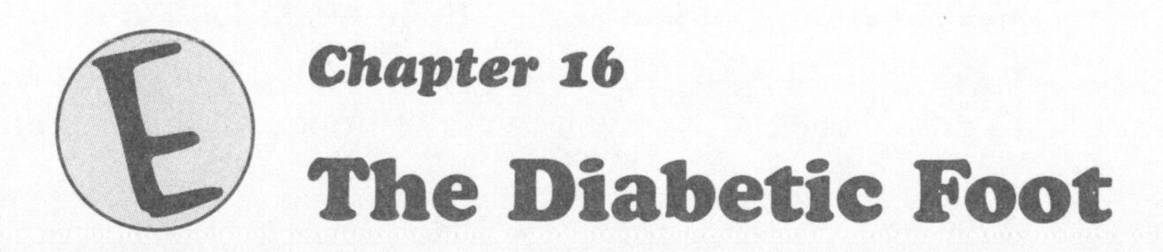

Chapter 16
The Diabetic Foot

What do your feet have to do with diabetes, you ask? A lot. Over time, high blood glucose levels can deaden your nerves and clog up the cardiovascular system, making neuropathy and peripheral vascular disease a real danger to the feet. And as someone with diabetes, your body is slower to heal and prone to infection, so small blisters and abrasions can quickly turn into serious complications if not treated promptly and properly.

Treat Your Feet Right

The American Podiatric Medical Association estimates that the average person walks about 115,000 miles in a lifetime (over four times around the equator, if you're counting). With all that walking, your feet get put through a lot of wear and tear. For most people, the pain of a blister or cut is a signal to get off your feet and let them heal. But if you have diabetic neuropathy (nerve damage) in your feet, the pain signal is impaired or gone altogether, and you may not notice an injury until you actually see it.

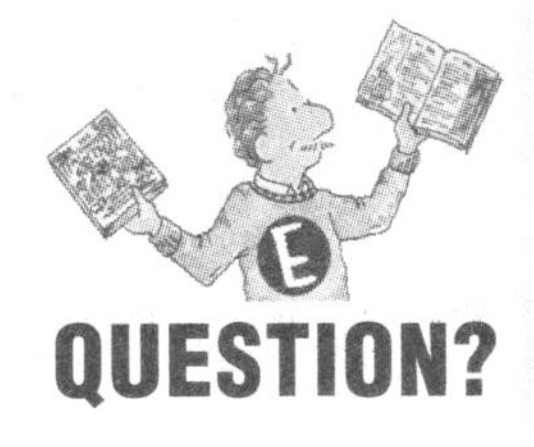

QUESTION?

My twelve-year-old daughter has type 1 diabetes. Do we really have to worry about her feet at such a young age?
While children and teens with type 1 are less likely to develop foot problems than adults, proper foot care is a good habit to get into early. As they grow older, nerve and circulatory impairment will become a bigger risk. In general, people with type 2 diabetes are at greater risk for foot complications simply because they often have extended periods of uncontrolled hyperglycemia before diagnosis.

Daily Foot Check

It only takes a minute to check your feet for signs of abrasions, blisters, or other problems, and it could save you serious medical problems down the road. Make it a part of your daily routine, either as you get dressed for the day, at shower time, or as you get ready for bed. Before you know it, it will become a healthy habit.

You should give your entire foot the once-over, and check between your toes. If you have flexibility and/or vision problems and have trouble seeing everything adequately, ask a family member for help. A flexible, magnified mirror can help you see those hard-to-reach spots.

Blisters, Corns, and Calluses

Do not pop or break blisters, as it will increase your risk of infection. Keep a close eye on the wounds. If they start to get worse, exhibit signs of infection (like pus, redness and warmth, or odor), or don't look as if they are healing within a day or so, call your doctor immediately for further instruction.

Keep your feet moisturized to avoid skin fissures or cracks caused by dryness. Try not to apply lotion between the toes, as it can breed fungal growth or infection. Instead, sprinkle baby or talcum powder to keep these areas dry. Peripheral neuropathy can cause a 10 percent decrease in skin moisture in the feet, so if you have any degree of PN, take extra care to use skin cream regularly.

If you develop corns or calluses, you're better off letting your podiatrist treat them. If you have PN, do *not* try to remove corns or calluses with cutting implements or chemical treatments on your own. A pumice stone may be used only with your doctor's approval.

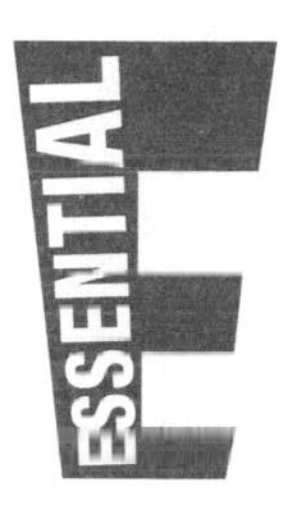

If you must soak in a tub or footbath, only use lukewarm water and make it brief. If you have any degree of neuropathy, you could unknowingly burn yourself. When you're done, dry your feet thoroughly with a thick towel, paying special attention to between your toes. Soaking is never recommended if you have an ulcer or foot wound.

Clipping Correctly

To prevent ingrown toenails, clip your nails straight across. Don't cut too close to the skin line to avoid an accidental slice into your skin. You can smooth out any sharp corners with an emery board. Thick or discolored toenails should be checked out by your podiatrist, as they could be a sign of a fungal infection.

The Right Equipment

Keeping your feet in good condition means proper protection against the elements. The only time you should be going barefoot is in bed and in the shower. Make sure your shoes and socks are appropriate for your needs.

An extra investment may be required, but in the long run the comfort and reduced risk of complications will be well worth the added expense.

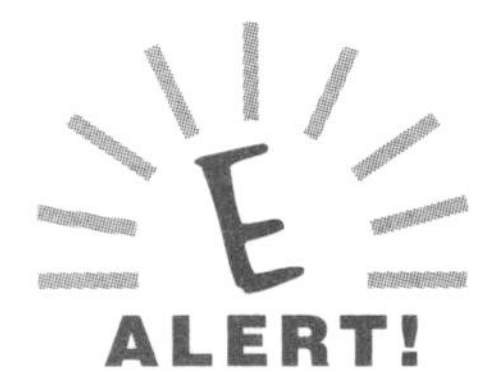

Invest in a pair of aqua socks or surf shoes if you visit the beach. The sand can be full of hidden hazards like broken glass and sharp seashells, and on a hot day the possibility of burning your feet is a real danger. Never go without foot protection in the water either.

Shoes Off the Rack

You have several options for shoes, ranging from regular, off-the-rack footwear to custom-made prescription shoes. If you don't have any diagnosed podiatric conditions, you can probably fulfill your footwear needs at a regular shoe store. However, there are some sensible shoe tips you should follow to keep your feet safe:

- **Stay grounded.** High heels are not good for your feet and can cause blisters.
- **On your toes.** Open-toed shoes also present a hazard, as they leave a good portion of your foot exposed. Skip the sandals and stay safe.
- **Get fit.** If at all possible, have a trained sales person check the fit of your shoes in the store.
- **Wiggle room.** Properly fitting shoes should leave room for your toes to move freely, and be wide and long enough for a firm yet comfortable fit.
- **Breathing room.** Leather or canvas uppers are your best bet for shoes that allow your feet to breathe, not sweat.

Shoes by Prescription

If you have existing foot problems, you'll probably need something a little more customized. Depth shoes are special therapeutic footwear that have extra room for the toes and for any orthotic inserts. If you have foot problems like hammertoes or bunions, depth shoes may be appropriate for you.

Orthotics are prescription devices that are inserted into shoes to relieve pressure and provide extra cushion and support. To produce a custom fit, your podiatrist may take special casts of your feet. Some newer orthotics production technology uses a sensor mat that you walk on to provide a computer-generated view of what portions of your feet bear the greatest load. Special software then designs the specifications for orthotics that are made to order. Your podiatrist or a specialist called an orthotist or pedorthist (a person trained in the design, fabrication, and fit of orthotic inserts) can help fit you for orthotics.

Health insurance frequently covers the cost of prescription footwear or devices, so check with your carrier. Medicare (Part B) covers 80 percent of the cost of depth-inlay shoes, custom-molded shoes, and shoe inserts for people with diabetes whose doctors certify that they meet clinical qualifications. Your podiatrist can tell you more about your coverage.

Custom-molded shoes may be required for some people with diabetes-related foot deformities such as cases of Charcot foot. Again, these customized shoes are obtained through a podiatrist or orthotist, who performs a special casting to fit the shoes properly.

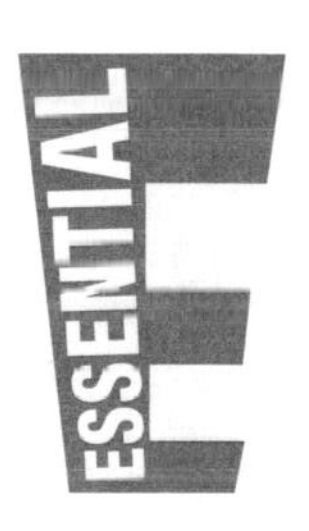

Comfort should be a prerequisite for any new pair of shoes you purchase. However, it's still a good idea to break them in gradually to avoid blisters. Wear them around the house for a short period daily for about a week until they start to feel "lived in."

Sock Sense

Even the best-fitting shoes won't do much good if you're wearing threadbare or hole-riddled socks. Lay a good foundation with thick, well-cushioned socks that are seamless (to prevent any friction blisters) and wick moisture away from the foot. Cotton, cotton-polyester, or acrylic blends are all good choices. There are also some newer treated fabrics and blends out on the market, like Teflon and antimicrobial fibers, designed to prevent blisters and infection. Since socks are a relatively small investment, it's a good idea to try out a variety until you find a type that suits you in style and comfort.

Tight and restrictive elastic bands (such as those on hosiery) can cut off circulation, but some degree of compression built in to the sock construction can be supportive and help to protect against deep-vein thrombosis. Other people, particularly those with edema (swollen feet), may do better with a loose-fitting sock. Your podiatrist can advise you on what's right for your particular needs.

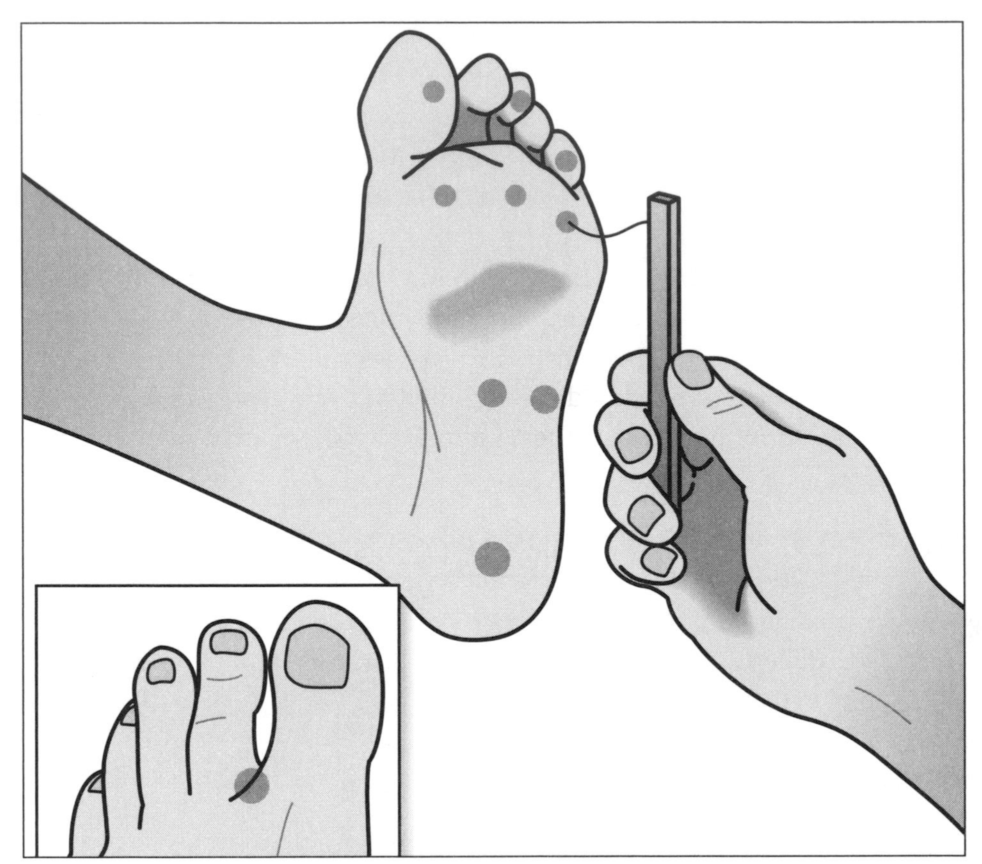

▲ The monofilament test for peripheral neuropathy.

Monofilament Test

Peripheral neuropathy (PN), or nerve damage of the extremities, is one of the most common complications of diabetes (60 percent of all people with the disease develop it at some point). Symptoms include burning, tingling, numbness, a prickly sensation (like "pins and needles"), and muscle weakness. Neuropathy is the result of chronically high blood sugars, so the best way to prevent it is to maintain good glucose control.

To check for neuropathy, your doctor should perform a monofilament test—a measure of the sensation in your feet—at least annually. In this simple yet sensitive evaluation, the monofilament, which is a piece of plastic fiber resembling fishing line, is touched against various parts of the sole of your foot, and your ability to feel it at varying pressure is assessed. It is sometimes called the 10-gram monofilament test because the fiber is calibrated to bend to 10 grams of pressure.

Your doctor may also use a tuning fork on the bottoms of your feet to see if you can sense the vibration. Nerve-conduction studies or velocity tests, which use electrodes to stimulate nerves and then measure the resulting impulses, are a less-frequently used, more sophisticated method of diagnosing some neuropathies. Electromyography (EMG), which uses thin needles inserted into the muscles to measure electrical impulses, may also be prescribed. These latter two tests can be painful, and may not be ordered unless there is some question about the diagnosis.

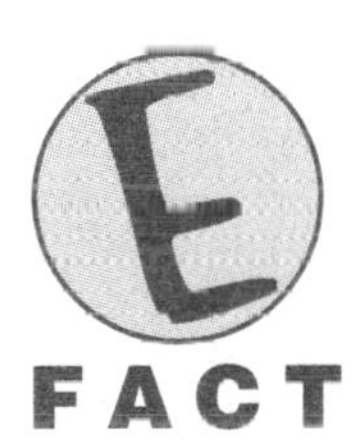

FACT

Avoid the use of hot-water bottles, heating pads, and other foot-warming devices if you have neuropathy. You could inadvertently burn yourself, so stick with a warm pair of socks. And never go without at least a pair of slippers on, even for a late-night trek to the bathroom, as you run the risk of tripping and injuring your exposed foot.

When to See a Podiatrist

For people with neuropathy, the ADA recommends a thorough foot exam at least annually and a visual inspection of the feet at each regular physician's appointment. Your regular doctor may perform these tests, or she may refer you to a podiatrist. A doctor of podiatric medicine (DPM) is a medical doctor with specialized training in the physiology and medical care of the foot and ankle. Podiatrists are licensed in all fifty states.

If you have diagnosed structural, nerve, or skin problems with your feet, a podiatrist should be on your diabetes care team, and you should see him every three to six months. Foot ulcers, in particular, require specialized wound care to avoid infection and possible amputation.

In addition to the regular tests for neuropathy described previously, a podiatrist will assess the pulse and blood pressure of the foot and ankle and the temperature of your feet to screen for circulatory problems. Ultrasound or Doppler may be used to check blood flow.

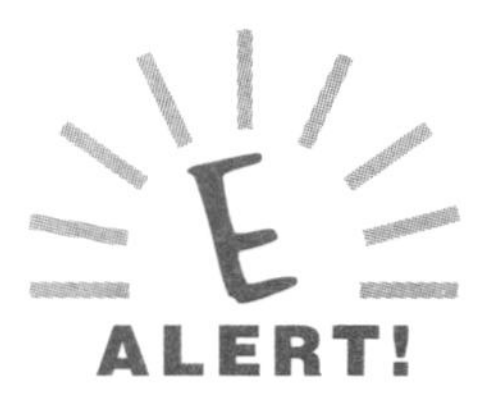

Add diabetic foot problems to the long list of negative health effects from smoking. Smoking tobacco constricts your blood vessels, which can make circulatory problems worse and restrict blood flow to your feet.

Charcot Foot or Joint

Charcot foot or joint, also called neuropathic arthropathy, is a podiatric condition that occurs in an estimated 9 to 30 percent of people suffering from diabetic peripheral neuropathy. It is caused by a breakdown of the joints and bones that goes unnoticed because of nerve damage and results in deformities of the bones of the feet. The condition is usually treated by a podiatrist or an orthopedist.

Typical signs of Charcot foot include extreme swelling, warmth of the skin, and redness. Since these are also signs of infection, cellulitis, or deep-vein thrombosis, x-ray examination is needed to confirm the diagnosis.

The Healing Process

In order to heal properly, a Charcot foot is usually immobilized in a contact cast, which is replaced periodically in order to inspect the foot. This foot-to-upper-leg cast cushions and protects the foot, and in many cases you may be able to walk on it with the help of crutches or a cane. However, some patients may be instructed to stay off their feet completely.

The cast may need to stay on as long as six months while the foot heals; after it is removed a leg brace may be required. Frequently, pressure ulcers form as a result of the foot deformity and consequent redistribution of weight. Reconstructive surgery may be required in extreme cases where ulcers become a recurring problem. Physical therapy can also help you regain motion and learn adaptive exercise techniques.

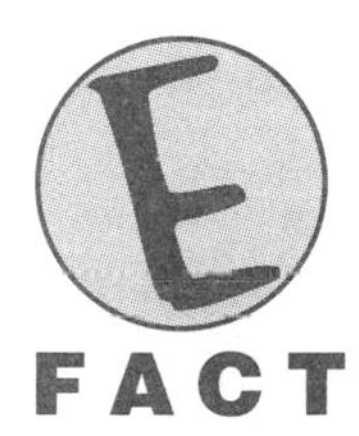
FACT

Diabetes is the leading cause of lower-extremity amputation in the United States, but at least half of all amputations could be prevented with early intervention and proper foot and skin care.

Diabetic Foot Ulcers

If you've ever had a shot of Novocain at the dentist, you know how it feels to try to talk or eat afterward—kind of like knitting with boxing gloves on. People who have lost the sensation in their feet have a similar experience. Neuropathy often causes an unnatural and awkward stride, which puts repeated pressure on the same spot of your foot. Over time, this area will callus and may eventually develop into a pressure ulcer. Other diabetic foot ulcers may be caused by poor circulation in your legs and feet. Beyond practicing good foot care, the best thing you can do to prevent limb-threatening complications from ulcers is detect them early and treat them properly.

How They Happen

Most ulcers form on the bottom of the foot, although shoes that don't fit well can cause sores and subsequent ulcers on the top of the foot or the ankle. Usually ulcers start as a callus, small sore, abrasion, or blister that would be "no big deal" in someone without diabetes. However, high blood glucose levels, poor circulation, and nerve damage are a recipe for ulceration in people with diabetes.

There are two categories of foot ulcers—vascular and neuropathic (or "pressure") ulcer. The former is caused by peripheral vascular disease; the latter is the result of the loss of sensation that accompanies peripheral neuropathy. People who have PN may put increased pressure on the same area of their foot repeatedly, resulting in callusing at first, and eventually in ulceration. Ulcers caused by PVD are usually painful, while those caused by PN are not.

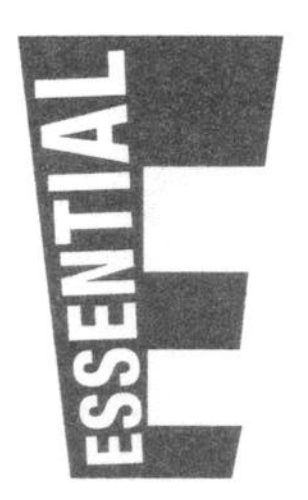

Keep those feet moving to ward off vascular ulcers and promote good circulation. Exercise (low-impact if you have foot problems), avoid sitting with your legs crossed for more than a few minutes at a time, and periodically stretch your legs and toes. Putting up your feet when you're at rest can also help blood flow.

Treatment

Infection is the primary risk with foot ulcers, so proper wound care is essential. Ulcers should remain moist and covered in a breathable dressing at all times (except when changing bandages). Oxygen is essential to the healing process. An antibiotic ointment may be applied if infection is present. Oral antibiotic medication should also be prescribed. If you have a pressure ulcer, debridement—removal of callused, dead skin—may also be performed at the podiatrist's office.

Your doctor may also prescribe one of several new "human-based" ulcer treatments, such as Apligraf (Organogenesis) and Regranex (Ortho-McNeil). Apligraf is a bioengineered tissue that contains skin cells and proteins, and Regranex is a gel containing platelet growth factors that promote healing and new skin growth.

Ulcers that are the result of PVD may show up on the lower leg as well as the foot. The toes are also a common location, and if circulation is poor enough, tissue necrosis (tissue death) or gangrene may be evident in the surrounding blackened skin. These patients may need an arterial bypass to restore blood flow to their feet and legs.

Osteomyelitis, or bone infection, may occur if infection in the ulcer spreads deeply enough. This is usually diagnosed with a bone scan or magnetic resonance imaging (MRI) and treated with intravenous antibiotic therapy.

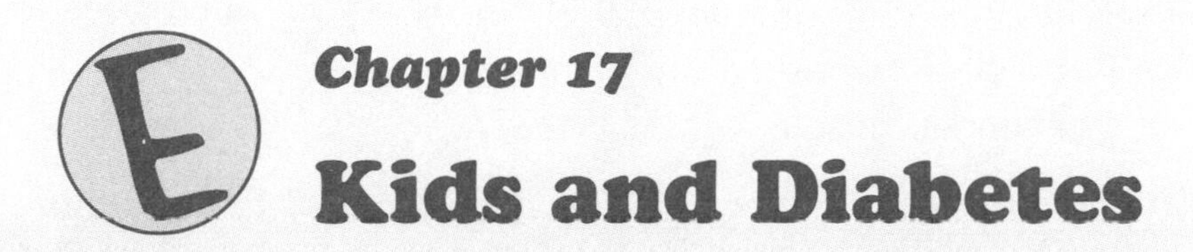

Chapter 17
Kids and Diabetes

Growing up with diabetes is a challenge for both child and parent. Dealing with doctors, bloodwork, school issues, medical supplies, and everything else that comes with the diabetes package is a full-time job in itself. But as your child grows, you'll find her taking more responsibility for her own care.

The Littlest Patients: Infants and Toddlers

As any parent can attest, not knowing how to help your hurting child is a horrible feeling. When your very young child has diabetes, she can't tell you if she's "feeling low" or needs to check her blood glucose. But just as parents develop a sense of a "hungry cry" versus a "wet cry," you will become attuned to the signs your child gives about how she's feeling.

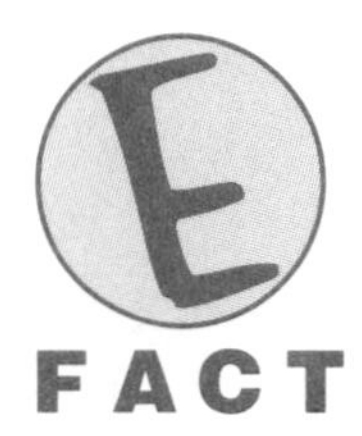

FACT

A pediatric endocrinologist is a physician trained to deal with endocrine disorders, such as diabetes, in children. If your child's pediatrician or general practitioner has little experience with children with type 1 diabetes, it's a good idea to get a pediatric endocrinologist on board for her treatment.

Recognizing Signs and Symptoms

The same symptoms that occur in older kids and adults signaling the possibility of type 1 diabetes apply to infants and toddlers; the difference is that since their verbal communication skills are limited, you probably won't recognize them as quickly. In addition, symptoms like fatigue are hard to discern in a baby who sleeps a good deal of the day anyway. The positive news is that most parents, particularly new ones, will take a "rather safe than sorry" attitude and take an inconsolable infant or toddler to the doctor to figure out what's wrong quickly rather than waiting around for things to worsen.

If your child is at risk for type 1 diabetes, you can be on the lookout for the following symptoms:

- Excessive wet diapers.
- Diaper rash that doesn't resolve quickly or keeps recurring.
- Constant hunger and/or thirst.
- Irritability or fussiness that doesn't seem related to colic.
- Sleeping more than usual.

Detecting Highs and Lows

Recognizing blood sugar highs and lows may be hard when a diabetes diagnosis is new in your very young child. Fortunately you have the best tool for making sure things are in balance right at your fingertips—a glucose monitor. If your child is acting the least bit out of sorts, always check glucose levels first. It may not be her diabetes, but if it is you want to find out quickly and treat it fast. Talk to your child's doctor about an appropriate amount of carbohydrates to treat her lows. As a general rule, kids under age six require 5 to 10 grams of a fast-acting carb if their blood glucose is low.

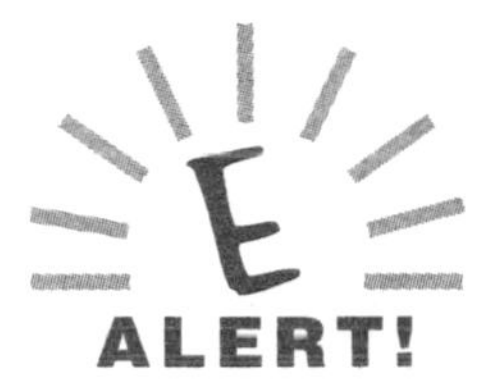

If you have an infant or toddler with diabetes, have an oral syringe on hand to administer a fast-acting liquid carb like syrup if a hypo occurs and your baby refuses a bottle of juice. Cake frosting in a tube and glucose gel can also work for more cooperative eaters. Never feed a child who has lost consciousness because of the risk of choking or aspiration, and never give an infant a glucose tablet or hard candy.

Glucose Monitoring

Glucose checks are a tough job for parents, especially in very young children who don't have the capacity to understand why they must get poked and prodded. You can make it a little easier by buying an alternate site meter, which allows you to test on less-sensitive areas like the forearm. You may also be able to stick the heel instead of the fingers. Talk to your child's doctor for her or his specific recommendations, and try out different meters until you find one that works well for you. Both you and your child will eventually get used to testing.

On Eating and Insulin

Small children have notoriously unpredictable appetites. They can go for days eating very little, and then suddenly down a whole plate of mac and cheese in the blink of an eye. Of course, if you don't know what your child is going to wolf down, or push away, at the next meal, it makes giving insulin a tad difficult. For this reason, your doctor may recommend rapid-acting insulin to be administered immediately following a meal to correctly cover the carbs and avoid highs or lows.

Insulin injections can be traumatic for young children, but there are several injection aids available to make the job easier on both of you. Your doctor can prescribe a topical anesthetic cream to numb the injection site, and a device called an Inject-Ease can be used with a standard syringe to both hide the needle and minimize pain by facilitating a rapid injection.

Taking Diabetes to School

Sending your child off to school for the first time is particularly tough for parents. In addition to all the usual parental worries, you have your child's diabetes to think about. The good news is that many, many others have gone before you and have blazed the trail, so to speak, for your child's rights in the classroom. If you face an uncooperative school staff, there are specific legal protections in place to ensure that your child gets appropriate medical care and fair, nondiscriminatory treatment while in the classroom.

Dealing with Discrimination

Every child will probably have to deal with some form of discrimination in his or her life, usually due to an ignorance of what type 1 diabetes is all about. It can be as simple as denying a child a cookie in the cafeteria, or as overt as denying self-monitoring for a child who is capable of performing it.

If your child goes to a public school or a private school that receives federal funding, she has specific educational rights under several federal laws. Section 504 of the Rehabilitation Act of 1973 allows you to develop two important documents that ensure your child's medical needs are met while she is at school—a Section 504 plan and an individualized education plan (IEP). A Section 504 plan outlines a child's basic medical needs (e.g., a source of fast-acting glucose if she is low), while the IEP outlines the specific actions your child should be able to take in light of the 504 (e.g., free access to her locker or bag to treat a low and the right to eat in the classroom if needed).

To qualify under Section 504, you need to provide a record of medical impairment, which can easily be provided by your child's physician. You also need to prove that if not treated effectively, diabetes can affect your child's educational performance, again something your doctor can verify.

Along with the Americans with Disabilities Act (ADA) and the Individuals with Disabilities Education Act (IDEA) of 1991, Section 504 also ensures that your child isn't unnecessarily restricted from participating fully in activities she is capable of joining, such as school sports, and that things like diabetes-related absences don't negatively impact her school record.

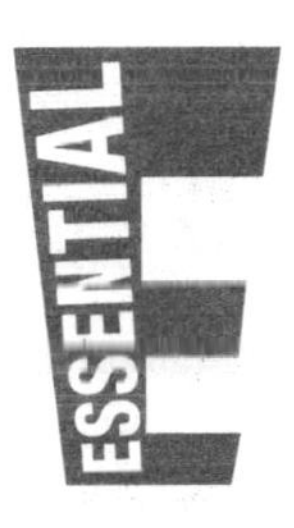

A federally funded school cannot legally refuse to administer medication to your child. In fact, they could lose their funding if they do so. If you have problems with your school or school district complying with your child's IEP, the American Diabetes Association is a great place to turn to for advocacy and support. Contact the ADA to find out your options.

A Section 504 IEP should cover at least the following areas:

- **Blood glucose monitoring requirements.** Spell out how often checks should occur, under what circumstances extra checks might be required (i.e., exercise), logging procedures, and how the meter and supplies should be stored.
- **Insulin requirements.** List insulin doses, when they should be taken, how much insulin is required for specific glucose values or for covering a meal, and how to properly store insulin. If your child uses an insulin pump, include information on that as well.
- **Meals, snacks, and fluids.** A dietary plan for meals eaten at school should describe your child's recommended carb intake for lunch and

snacks, when he or she should eat, and also how to handle special occasions (i.e., birthday cakes at school).

- **Recognizing and treating highs and lows.** The plan should explain the signs of both hypoglycemia (low blood glucose) and hyperglycemia (high blood glucose), and how to promptly and correctly treat both. Explicit directions on the administration of a glucagon shot should also be included, and staff should be trained in its use as well.
- **Ketone testing.** Explain when ketone testing is appropriate and how the procedure works.
- **Contact information.** This probably goes without saying, but make sure your IEP includes your full contact information, a backup emergency contact, and a backup for your backup. Someone should be reachable at all times.

Educating the Educators

If your child goes to a school that receives federal funding, the school itself is legally required to provide necessary diabetes training to educators and other personnel. However, it's in your best interest to get involved in the process early on. Ask to attend any teaching sessions the school sets up to ensure their accuracy and provide practical input on how the information specifically applies to your child.

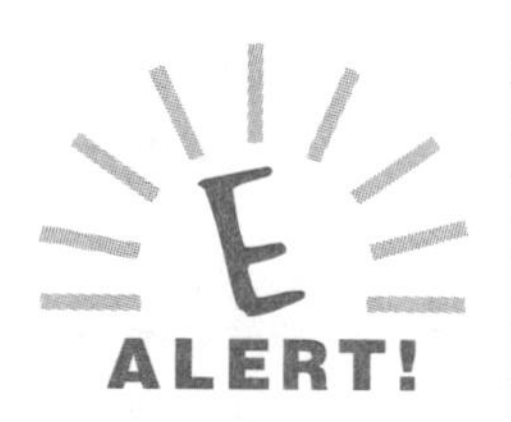

If your child's school has a nurse on duty who will help your child with his diabetes care, schedule a meeting with her to go over your child's particular treatment needs and to ensure that she knows exactly what to do in case of a hypoglycemic emergency. The nurse should also attend any diabetes training sessions.

Your child's school may ask you for input or assistance in coordinating teacher training. This is a good opportunity to get your diabetes educator in to meet with all the teaching staff and support personnel (i.e., bus driver, cafeteria workers, playground personnel) that your child will have contact with in order to make them aware of her medical needs and to provide them with an accurate, working knowledge of what type 1 diabetes is really all about.

School personnel who have contact with your child should be trained in all aspects of diabetes care. Even the most competent child may have situations where his blood glucose drops too low and he needs assistance with a check and/or a quick fix of glucose.

Treatment in the Classroom

Your child's school is not legally obligated to allow blood glucose testing in the classroom, and your son or daughter may be required to go to the nurse's office or another place to check glucose levels. However, for older children who are both capable of doing a check themselves and comfortable with doing it in class, it is usually in the best interest of all involved if the child is allowed to do checks right in the classroom. Your child will miss less class time—if they are feeling low they don't have to use up precious time traveling to the nurse's office—and it is less disruptive to the entire class if they can discretely check without leaving the room.

There should always be a fast-acting glucose snack available in your child's classroom for her immediate use. You will have primary responsibility for keeping an adequate supply available for her, as well as keeping unexpired meter strips and supplies, insulin, and everything else she needs in stock. The school should have a separate, dedicated meter for her use, along with a separate logbook she can use to record results. Request to have a photocopy of your child's readings sent home with her at the end of each day.

School Sports

Sports are another area where children may be treated differently because they have diabetes. Kids who want to get involved with team or individual sports should not be dissuaded or automatically excluded on the basis of their diabetes alone. With appropriate precautions, your child can excel in just about anything she wishes.

If your child is participating in school sports, her coach should be involved in diabetes training along with other educators. It's particularly important that coaches realize the signs of hypoglycemia, since exercise may induce a low, and know how to treat it appropriately.

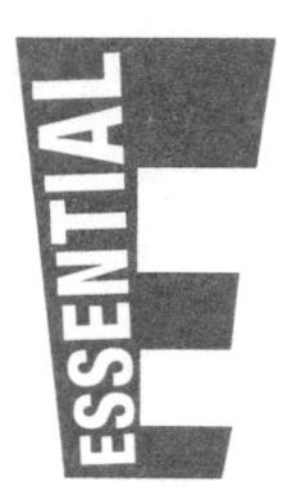

Coaches or instructors of team or individual sports that take place outside of the school setting also need proper education about your child's medical needs. If you can, consider volunteering to coach or help out with the team to make the learning curve a little easier.

Coming of Age with Diabetes

The preteen and teen years are a rocky time for all kids, as their social identities emerge, they start such eternally awkward rituals as dating, and they pull away from their parents to find their own sense of self and establish their independence. This is a particularly tricky time for adolescents with diabetes, who may be desperately trying to find a way to "fit in" when their blood glucose checks, insulin pump, and eating habits all say—"I'm different."

The hormonal changes of puberty also take a toll on diabetes control in and of themselves, increasing overall insulin resistance. Girls and boys face a sea change in their bodies that makes control a bit more elusive than normal. Things will stabilize after a time. (For more on dealing with puberty see Chapters 18 and 19.)

This is also an age for experimentation with drugs, alcohol, and smoking, all things that will affect your child's blood glucose control in ways he or she is not accustomed to. Worse, drugs and alcohol can impact your child's perception of blood glucose lows and impair his ability to make good decisions. Now is the time to have a frank talk about drugs, alcohol, and cigarettes. Your child needs to know how it will affect his diabetes, and what precautions he needs to take if he does try any of these things. Giving him this information is not the same as saying you approve of his experimentation with drugs or alcohol; in fact, he also needs to know explicitly that you don't want him using at all. But since adolescence is often filled with bad decisions as teens try to find their own identity, educating your child for the possibility could literally save his life.

Sex is another area where a candid discussion is necessary. Your adolescent needs to know about birth control, and the risks of unprotected sex in terms of sexually transmitted diseases and unwanted pregnancy. Again, you don't have to condone it, but you do need to provide vital information.

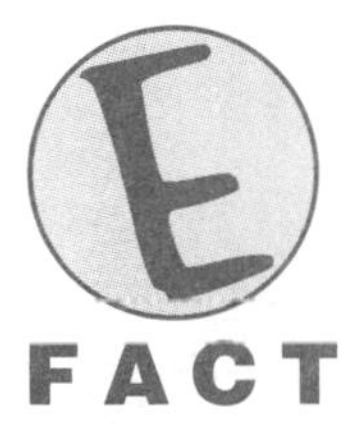

A full explanation of the risks both mother and child face during pregnancy when blood glucose levels are not well controlled is in order. Keep it balanced. Make sure your teen recognizes that when she is older and ready to start a family, a safe and healthy *planned* pregnancy is achievable.

Handling Special Days

Birthdays, slumber parties, Halloween—sometimes it seems like childhood is one big food fest. It's hard to deny your child special treats when all her peers are digging in. Fortunately, with insulin adjustments and good planning, your child can partake in some of the sweet treats of childhood in moderation.

Happy Halloween!

As the only holiday devoted almost exclusively to gorging on sugar-laden treats, Halloween holds a special place in hell for most parents dealing with diabetes. This can understandably be a very tough time for your child to get through, but you can make it easier. Try focusing on the real spirit of the season and make a special haunted house for the kids, or let them have a spooktacular party with ghost stories, rubber spiders, and the old "spaghetti intestines and grape eyeballs" game. For younger kids, a costume party with pumpkin painting and other activities is always fun. If you're hosting, you can control the quality and quantity of snacks.

You can also make a game of trading small toys, books, stickers, and nonedible prizes with your kids for their sweet loot. Make each item worth a certain number of candy pieces, and they can brush up on their math skills as well. Know the carb counts of the fun-sized treats and be the gatekeeper for the candy they do keep.

Birthday Parties

When a birthday invitation arrives, talk to the host parent ahead of time to find out what's on the menu. If it's something your child is particularly sensitive to, bring a special snack. Make sure the parent knows what amount of cake and/or ice cream is allowed. You may have to accompany your child to most parties, even when he surpasses the age where most parents hang around. With a full list of other guests to attend to, you can't reasonably expect the party hosts to attend to your child's medical needs, especially if the birthday child is a classroom acquaintance and the parents are largely unfamiliar with diabetes and your child's special needs.

If attending the party becomes an issue with your child and her growing sense of independence, assure her that you'll fade into the background as much as possible except when your help is needed. When the celebration takes place at a public venue like a skating rink or a movie theater, this is a bit easier on both of you. Think about bringing siblings and making a separate family affair out of it so you're almost not even there. This usually works out best for all involved—you aren't hanging around, making your child feel self-conscious, it gives the host parent peace of mind to know you are in the area should your help be needed, and you feel better knowing your child is nearby. Your other kids and/or your spouse also get a day of fun out of it, so everyone wins.

Overnight Trips

The first solo sleepover can be nerve-wracking for both you and the host parents. Kids old enough for slumber parties and overnight trips are typically at least starting to manage some of their own diabetes care, which helps. Spend some time with the parents in advance of the event to give them a briefing on what your child might potentially need, and make yourself available via phone for any questions they might have during the visit. Provide them with a one-page sheet with all treatment basics; trouble signs will be helpful as well.

Finding Baby Sitters

Caring for a child with chronic illness takes a big emotional and physical toll on parents, and you, too, need an occasional break from it all. It's true that caregivers, especially for small children with diabetes, can be difficult to find. Some adults feel overwhelmed by the responsibility of caring for a child (think about how you felt when your child was first diagnosed). Others worry about legal liability should something go wrong under their care. Fear is a big factor in many people's unwillingness to baby-sit children with diabetes, and this is often the easiest obstacle to overcome.

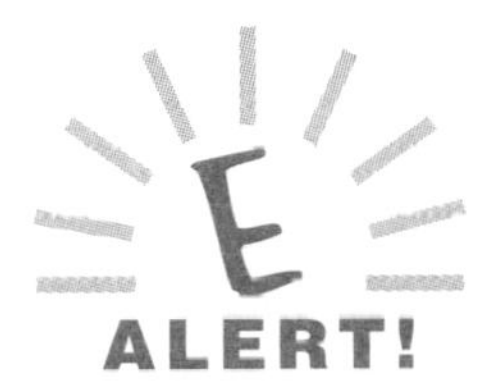

Don't give up on finding a baby sitter out of hand because you've been unsuccessful before. And don't stay with your child constantly because you live in fear of the worst possible scenario happening when you're away.

If you have relatives nearby, they are a natural choice for baby-sitting duties. If not, tap friends and neighbors for potential candidates. You need someone responsible, caring, and cool-headed—the same qualities you would look for in a baby sitter if your child didn't have diabetes. When you make first contact, explain up front that your child does have diabetes and has some special needs. Then invite your potential sitter over for an afternoon (or even several afternoons) to interact and watch your child with you around as backup, to see what caring for your child really entails. Often the sitter will find that the reality is not even close to what his imagination had cooked up.

When you leave your child with a sitter, always leave a list of emergency contact numbers (including your child's doctor's office), along with detailed instructions on your child's diabetes care. If you have an extra copy of your child's IEP around, photocopying it for sitters is a good idea since it contains all essential treatment information.

Kids Being Kids

Children with diabetes who live in rural areas often are the only child in their school or possibly even their community who has to deal with the special issues related to living with this disease. Even children in more populated areas can sometimes feel alone and isolated, as can their parents.

What about Diabetes Camp?

Diabetes camp can be a great adventure for children—teaching them management skills that will last a lifetime and, equally as important, giving them the chance to spend a few weeks with peers who share their concerns and experiences. There are diabetes camp programs across the United States; Appendix A lists some resources for finding a camp near you. Most are, of course, summer programs, and many of the counselors at these camps also have diabetes and can relate to your children as a mentor and a diabetes peer and/or role model. In addition to all the typical summer camp activities like swimming, canoeing, and crafts, your child will learn more about her or his diabetes and how to care for it.

Finally, you can have a care-giving respite with the peace of mind that your child is someplace where you know his or her diabetes will be well taken care of.

Type 2 and Kids—A Growing Problem

A 2002 study on obesity and children in the *New England Journal of Medicine* brought to light the growing problem of kids, weight, and insulin resistance, finding a strong association between childhood obesity and impaired glucose tolerance. According to the U.S. Department of Health and Human Services, the percentage of newly diagnosed children who are classified as having type 2 diabetes has climbed from less than 5 percent before 1994 to 30 to 50 percent in subsequent years.

In addition, the number of overweight children overall is increasing at an alarming rate—5.3 million, or 12.5 percent, of Americans between ages six and seventeen are considered obese. Aside from type 2 diabetes, childhood obesity can lead to adult medical issues like atherosclerosis, hypertension, respiratory infections, and sleep apnea.

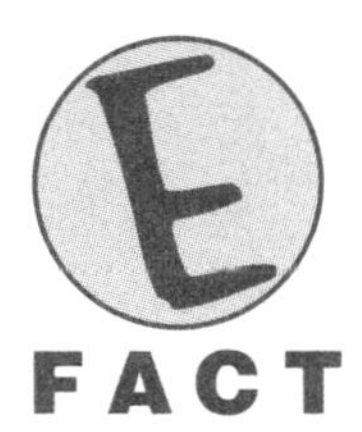
FACT

Studies show that sugary sweet soft drinks can increase the likelihood of a child becoming obese by up to 60 percent. The extra calories in sweet drinks such as Kool-Aid and sodas can cause significant weight gain if not consumed in moderation, so look to sugar-free or diet soda alternatives.

Weight Control and Exercise

If your child is at risk for developing type 2 diabetes and has issues with weight, diet and exercise should be your immediate defense plan. Your pediatrician can formulate a medically sound weight-loss program that is tailored to your child's specific needs. A registered dietitian can also be of great help in creating a balanced meal plan for your child.

Every child, no matter what her level of athleticism, should be encouraged to get out and get moving. If she's interested, sign her up for some team sports and/or outdoor activities. If she isn't into athletics, activities such as bike and scooter riding, in-line skating, hiking, swimming, or dancing are good, noncompetitive ways to get fit. The important thing is to find something that interests her so it becomes something she looks forward to instead of dreading.

Keep food itself in perspective and treat it as fuel, not entertainment, comfort, love, or reward. Using treats to make a child feel better instead of communicating about her problems turns food into an inappropriate substitute for affection, and can sabotage self-esteem and self-sufficiency.

Diabetes is a family disease, whether it be type 1 or type 2. Kids can't be expected to diet and exercise if their parents and siblings are living a fast-food, couch-potato lifestyle. Plan meals and group activities that everyone can enjoy together.

If your child has been diagnosed with type 2 diabetes, now is the time to get him on the path to healthy food attitudes and fitness to get both bad habits and his diabetes under control. What your child learns now will serve him well for the rest of his life.

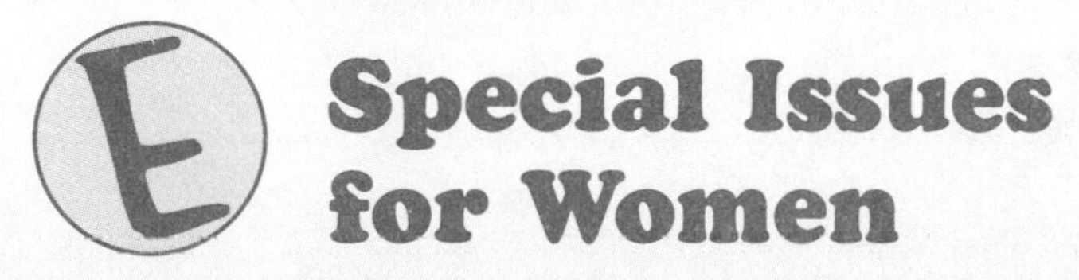

Chapter 18

Special Issues for Women

Feeling as if you're in a permanent state of PMS—even if you're well past menopause? The hormonal tides of puberty, pregnancy, menstruation, and menopause are each yet another seismic force to contend with as you try to maintain balance and control of your diabetes. Remember that treatment is not a static thing; "adapt, adapt, adapt" will be your motto as you move through the stages of diabetes care.

At Puberty

The barrage of hormones, social turmoil, fashion crises, and other adolescent dramas that spells puberty can also spell trouble for your teen's (or preteen's) diabetes control. Issues of poor self-image and of wanting to fit in with peers by acting and eating as they do may raise glucose levels, either through noncompliance with treatment or as a stress response. Hormonal changes, which magnify all of the preceding and can increase the need for insulin, compound the problem.

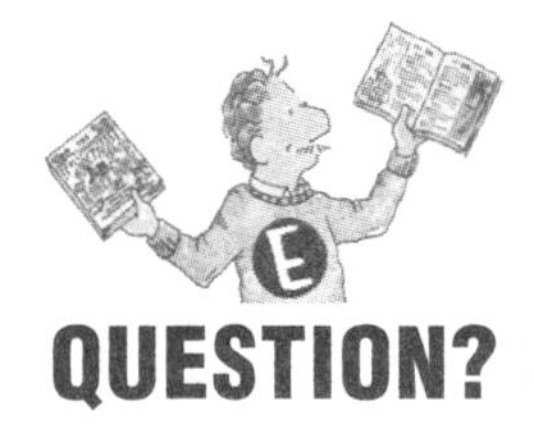

QUESTION?

I've heard skipping my insulin is an easy way to lose some weight. Can I do it if I don't eat much?

Skipping your shot can be deadly. While you might lose a little, DKA is a very real risk along with all the other hazards of poor control. Your body probably needs more insulin right now because of the hormonal changes of puberty. It's really important to talk to someone about how you're feeling. Start with your doctor—a good doc won't judge you or make you feel bad—she'll try to help.

Girls going through puberty will have an increased need for insulin as estrogen and progesterone production rev up with menarche (the first menstrual period). The peak age for type 1 diabetes diagnosis for girls is between the ages of ten and twelve, when puberty is often in full bloom.

At Risk for Eating Disorders

Eating disorders are more than twice as common in teenage girls with diabetes than those without. Girls with eating disorders may skip their insulin dosage–a practice called insulin omission–in an effort to lose weight. They are also at a higher risk for developing diabetic ketoacidosis (DKA) and poor overall control (as measured by A1c levels).

Diabetes and Menstruation

If you are a premenopausal woman with diabetes, you may notice a rise in blood glucose levels as your menstrual period draws closer. The rise in estrogen and progesterone levels that occurs toward the end of the cycle (about a week before menstruation) can increase insulin resistance, causing a rise in glucose levels. In other women with diabetes, this hormonal change may actually increase insulin sensitivity, triggering lower blood sugar levels. And in the true one-size-fits-none nature of diabetes, some women may experience no changes at all.

Tracking your glucose levels throughout your monthly cycle can help you understand if hormones are having an impact on your diabetes control (yet one more thing to keep in your blood glucose log). Discuss your results with your doctor. Adjustments in medication, insulin, exercise, and diet may be necessary to bring your glucose levels back to normal during this time.

Pregnancy: Treatment for Two

Having a baby is not a decision to be entered into lightly for anyone. For women with diabetes, the decision may be even more difficult because of the demands placed on their body, the necessity for painstaking control before and during the pregnancy, and the potential for developing or worsening diabetic complications in the process.

Some complications of diabetes, including retinopathy, nephropathy, and neuropathy, can get worse in pregnancy. Your doctor will counsel you about your specific risks as part of preconception planning. Tests that may be ordered during preconception planning include:

- Thyroid (TSH; for type 1)
- Kidney function (serum creatinine, twenty-four-hour urine)
- Comprehensive eye exam
- Cardiovascular screening

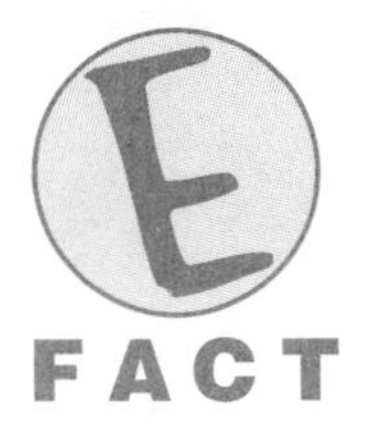

Diabetic retinopathy is one condition that pregnancy may make worse. The ADA recommends that in addition to a dilated-eye exam during preconception planning, women who become pregnant should have a comprehensive eye exam in the first trimester and close follow-up with an ophthalmologist throughout pregnancy if retinopathy is present.

Control Before Conception

When it comes to having a successful pregnancy with type 1 or type 2 diabetes, planning is everything. Achieving good blood glucose control before conception is the best way to ensure a good outcome for both you and your child. The ADA recommends that women who plan on becoming pregnant strive for an A1c level of less than 7 percent, and pre- and postprandial glucose readings as outlined in the following table.

Recommended Glucose Readings for Women Planning to Conceive

	Whole Blood	Plasma
Preprandial (before meals)	70–100 mg/dl (3.9–5.6 mmol/l)	80–110 mg/dl (4.4–6.1 mmol/l)
2 hour postprandial (after meals)	<140 mg/dl (<7.8 mmol/l)	<155 mg/dl (<8.6 mmol/l)

If you take drugs for hypertension or other diabetic complications, your doctor will discuss your options with you, as many are not recommended for pregnancy. Drug therapy that is contraindicated in pregnancy, including oral diabetes medications, will have to be stopped and replaced with insulin therapy (which is considered safe in pregnancy). Starting insulin before you try to conceive will give you the chance to become accustomed to the routine and make appropriate dosage adjustments for optimal control.

Ideally, blood glucose will be stabilized at the target goal, or as close as possible to it, for several months before you try to conceive.

Adjustments to insulin and other aspects of your treatment will probably have to be made during pregnancy, too, which is why it's important to continue to involve your endocrinologist or diabetes care specialist, as well as your ob-gyn, in your treatment throughout your pregnancy.

Staying Healthy During Pregnancy

Once you become pregnant, your provider may recommend that you see a perinatologist, an ob-gyn that specializes in high-risk pregnancies. As with any member of your diabetes care team, you should make sure the physician you choose communicates clearly and proactively with you and your other providers, answers your questions to your satisfaction, and encourages you to play an active role in your treatment.

Your insulin needs will probably go up in pregnancy, as your placenta starts to manufacture hormones that increase your insulin resistance. Frequent glucose checks during this time are critical, and your doctor may also administer A1c testing each month or every six weeks instead of the typical three-month interval.

Your Baby and Diabetes

Get your baby's doctor on board early. A neonatologist, a doctor who cares for newborns with special health needs, may be consulted to be in the delivery room at birth in case of any problems. Choosing a pediatrician early is also a good idea.

If you are able to keep your blood glucose well controlled during pregnancy, your baby's risk of complications is reduced dramatically. Tight control in the first trimester in particular is important, because this is the critical time when the organ systems are developing in the fetus.

Babies born to mothers with diabetes have a greater chance of being born large for birth weight. This is because the fetus converts extra glucose into body fat in the womb. The condition, called macrosomia, puts newborns at risk for unplanned C-section birth and shoulder dystocia (getting wedged in the birth canal during delivery).

When the hard work of active labor starts to kick in to high gear, your insulin needs will drop. This is, after all, the ultimate form of exercise. And just like a strenuous workout, you run the risk of going low. Your glucose levels will be tested regularly, and you may have an IV line or heparin lock inserted to infuse glucose or insulin for type 1 as needed. Talk to your ob-gyn or perinatologist well before your due date to discuss the protocol used to prevent hypos in labor.

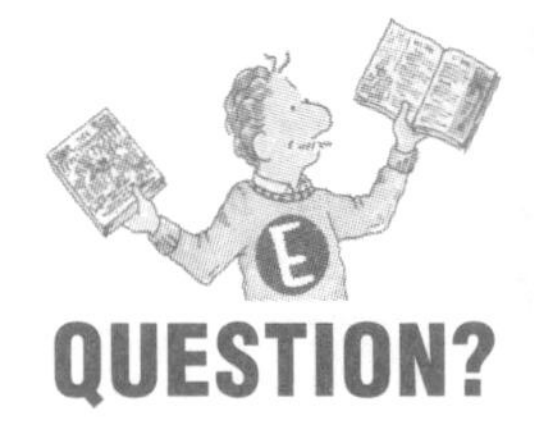

QUESTION?

I have had type 2 diabetes for five years, and my doctor just added a diagnosis of PCOS. Are they related?

Just like type 2 diabetes, polycystic ovary syndrome (PCOS) is characterized by insulin resistance. High cholesterol, hypertension, and heart disease are also hallmark symptoms. PCOS triggers an overabundance of androgens (male sex hormones) and too little estrogen, causing cysts to form in the ovaries.

Because of your medical history, your labor and delivery team will be on the lookout for hypoglycemia. While still in your womb, your baby's pancreas had been programmed to produce enough insulin to counteract your sometimes-heightened blood glucose supply. Once he becomes "disconnected" from the maternal sugar source at delivery, his high insulin levels may drive his blood glucose down, causing hypoglycemia. A heel stick blood test can confirm the diagnosis, and oral glucose or a glucose IV drip for baby can quickly treat the condition.

Having a parent with type 1 diabetes makes your child slightly more likely to develop the disease (2 to 5 percent; higher if another parent or sibling has the disease). Type 2 has a stronger genetic link, but the good news is it is easier to prevent with healthy lifestyle changes.

Breastfeeding

Many women with diabetes question their ability to breastfeed, worrying about either harm to their baby—Is my milk safe? Does it have enough nutrients?—or uncontrolled blood glucose swings in themselves—Will I go high from having to eat more? Will I go low from "sharing" with baby? You may be relieved to find out that women with diabetes can and do breastfeed successfully, and in fact your milk may even reduce the chances of passing diabetes on to baby.

Breast Benefits

Babies who breastfeed at least three months have a lower incidence of type 1 diabetes, and may be less likely to become obese as adults. And some research has linked early exposure to cow's milk and cow's milk–based formula to the development of type 1 diabetes, another good reason to nurse your child.

Clinical studies have also shown that women who have gestational diabetes in pregnancy and go on to breastfeed their child for at least three months experience improved pancreatic beta cell function, which may lessen their chances of developing type 2 diabetes later in life. Breastfeeding may also be protective for the children of at-risk type 2 populations. Several studies have shown that Native American mothers who breastfeed reduce the risk of their children developing the disease.

Safety Measures

Taking insulin does not threaten the health of your breastfeeding infant. However, women who take medication to control their type 2 diabetes need to consult with their doctor, as some drugs pass into breastmilk. Your doctor can help you weigh the benefits of breastfeeding against any risks medication might pose. In some cases, he may be able to prescribe an alternative drug. If you are pregnant and plan on breastfeeding your child, you should discuss these issues with your doctor now, so you are both prepared once baby arrives.

Breastfeeding can be hard work (especially for first-time moms), and when you're trying to balance it with the demanding occupation of new motherhood, the associated stress and fatigue can do a number on your control. The hormonal changes associated with breastfeeding and the postpartum period can also cause highs and lows (although in some women, this shift may improve sugar levels). As you may have guessed already, checking your glucose levels often and working with your doctor is the best way to stay on track during this hectic time.

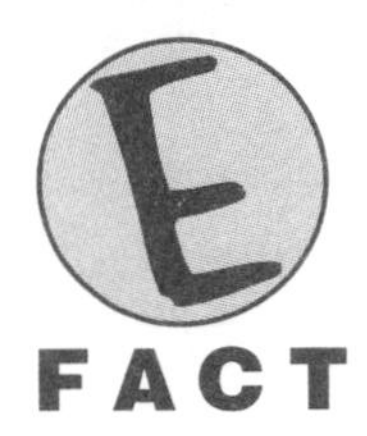

FACT

As with mothers without diabetes, there is no set timetable for weaning. However, when you and baby decide it is time, it should be done gradually if possible. In addition to stirring up the hormones again, you may have to adjust your diet to stay consistent with your control. Talk to your dietitian about your particular needs.

Avoiding Hypos

You'll need extra calories and fluid in your daily diet to keep your milk supply and your energy level up. If you haven't seen your dietitian lately, now's the time to go in for a refresher appointment. She can help you to create a meal plan that can promote successful breastfeeding, reasonable postpartum weight loss, and good diabetes control.

Not surprisingly, nursing can cause a drop in blood glucose levels. To avoid going low, have a protein/carb snack and something to drink either before or during nursing. This is particularly important for those middle-of-the-night feedings. Keep some quick and easy snacks on hand where you nurse, or consider setting up a minifridge with a childproof lock.

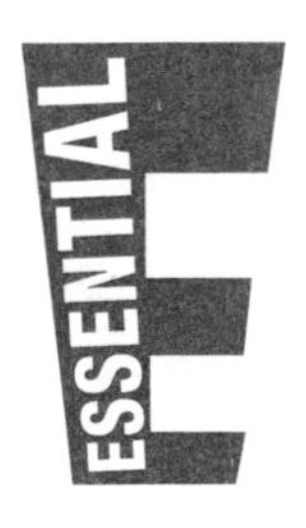

Glucose tablets or other fast-acting sugars should be easily accessible in case of a low, and a meter should be stowed within reach to make checking levels easy (but don't forget to store it more securely once baby is old enough to get around, which will be sooner than you think).

When It's Time for Menopause

The big change in your early fifties usually brings about changes in your diabetes treatment needs as well. In addition to the mood swings, the slowdown of estrogen and progesterone production can put your blood sugars on a swing of their own. In fact, you may actually start experiencing these symptoms well before menopause, in the preceding period known as perimenopause, which starts anywhere from age forty-five to fifty-five (average age being forty-seven).

How Menopause Affects Diabetes

Lower estrogen levels may increase insulin resistance in type 2 women, while lower progesterone levels have the opposite effect, increasing insulin sensitivity. For this reason, one woman's glycemic (or blood sugar) response to menopause can be very different from another's. The best way to figure out what's going on with you is to test your glucose levels frequently and work closely with your doctor.

On average, the ADA reports that most women require less medication (for blood glucose control) for type 2 diabetes after menopause. However, weight gain, which occurs in response to a slowing metabolism and declining estrogen levels, may offset this benefit, as can inactivity.

According to the Mayo Clinic, women with diabetes who are postmenopausal have a risk of heart attack or stroke that is three times that of their peers without diabetes.

HRT: Risks Versus Benefits

Whether or not to take hormone replacement therapy to combat some of the menopausal problems unique to women with diabetes is very much an individual decision, based on your own medical situation and cardiovascular risk profile. Oral estrogen therapy may improve your cholesterol profile by lowering your LDL (bad) and raising your HDL (good) cholesterol, but it has also been found to increase triglyceride levels, which ups cardiovascular risk. In fact, preliminary data released in 2002 from the Women's Health Initiative (WHI) trial found that HRT estrogen/ progestin therapy increased the risk of breast cancer, pulmonary embolism, and cardiovascular disease in postmenopausal women. The jury is still out on whether estrogen therapy alone carries similar health risks.

Female Sexual Dysfunction

In this post-Viagra age, the American public is well aware of the problems of male impotency. But female sexual dysfunction and arousal problems remain a less publicized cause. You may be surprised to learn that according to results of a national study published in the *Journal of the American Medical Association* in 1999, sexual dysfunction was actually more prevalent in women than in men (43 versus 31 percent).

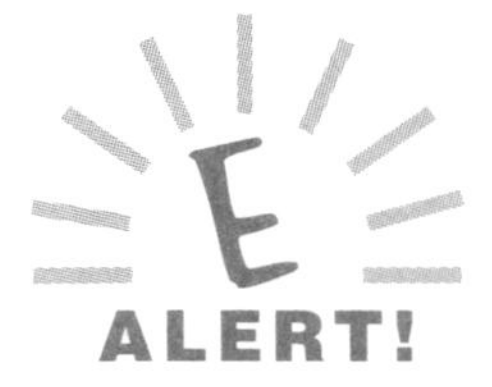

If you're suffering from sexual dysfunction, you need to talk to your care provider, or a gynecologist or urologist, about the problem. In some cases, it may be a sign of an underlying, undiagnosed diabetic complication that needs treatment. Even if it is something more benign, you owe it to yourself to find a solution. Don't let embarrassment stop you—your doctor is there to help.

Uncontrolled blood glucose levels affect arousal, performance, and overall well-being. High blood sugars trigger yeast infections and vaginal irritation. In addition, vascular damage can restrict blood flow to the vagina, causing lubrication problems. Women who have neuropathy that affects the genital area, the reproductive organs, and/or the vagina may have difficulty achieving arousal and orgasm.

Psychological Factors

Sometimes the problem is more psychological than physical. The less-romantic aspects of treatment, such as needing to do a blood sugar check before sex, can make some women self-conscious and less likely to initiate or participate in it.

Fear may be a factor in your ability to let go and relax, as well. You may be afraid that the physical exertion of sex will trigger hypoglycemia. Taking the same precautions you do for exercise will almost always prevent blood sugar lows. However, make sure your partner knows that in the unlikely event that you do lose consciousness, it wasn't his performance that did it. Give him a briefing on when to seek emergency medical care for you. Chapter 14 has more on hypoglycemia prevention and education.

Other Culprits

A number of other issues can contribute to sexual difficulties in women with diabetes. These include:

- Certain medications (e.g., antidepressants, hypertension medications)
- Menopause (low estrogen levels can cause vaginal dryness)
- Vaginismus (a tightening of the vaginal walls that may make sex painful)
- Excess weight or obesity—women who are overweight may feel self-conscious and unattractive

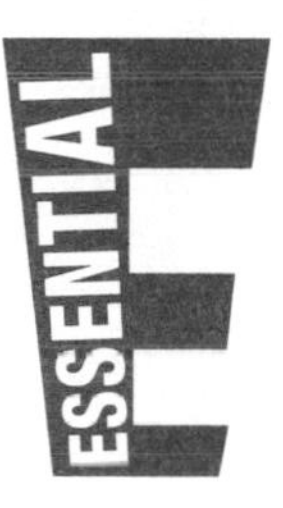

Wearing an insulin pump can present some unique challenges in the bedroom. If you decide you want to disconnect it before sex, be sure to take into account the amount of time you are off the pump and the exertion factor, and adjust accordingly once you're pumping again. If you prefer to stay hooked up, you may choose to use a longer infusion or tubing set.

Treatments

Therapy and/or medication may help you overcome depression. Make sure you talk to your doctor about the possible sexual side effects of any antidepressant she may prescribe. Some newer drugs, such as Wellbutrin (buproprion), have lower risks of sexual side effects and may be preferred.

If low estrogen levels are at the root of vaginal dryness problems, vaginal estrogen cream can sometimes alleviate this problem, but it should be prescribed with caution in some women. Over-the-counter lubricants are also available to ease dryness and painful penetration. And medical devices designed to stimulate blood flow in the genitals and increase lubrication may also be prescribed. Your gynecologist or urologist can tell you more about these options.

As with most complications related to diabetes, adjustments to your diet, medication, and exercise routines may improve both your diabetes and your sex drive.

How Women Cope

Managing chronic illness day in and day out can be stressful and emotionally draining. If you're newly diagnosed, you're trying to get your mental and physical bearings to figure out your own path to diabetes control. You've been thrown into this disease headfirst, and, even with the best diabetes care team guiding you, these early days can be stressful, scary, and anxious. In a worst-case scenario, you may have been handed a diagnosis, a one-size-fits-all "diabetic diet" and/or prescription, and shown the door to figure things out on your own (if such is the case, Chapter 5 can give you some advice on hiring a capable care team who won't leave you hanging).

Dealing with Depression

People with diabetes are up to three times more likely to suffer from depression than the general population, and women with diabetes are more likely to experience depression than men. It's normal to experience some depressive symptoms at diagnosis, but when depression starts to interfere with everyday life and you start to lose interest in things you used to enjoy, you may be experiencing a major depressive episode.

Depression distracts you from proper diabetes care, and clinical studies have shown that people with diabetes who are depressed have higher blood glucose levels and a higher incidence of microvascular and macrovascular diabetic complications. Add poor control, and the symptoms and psychological impact of knowing you aren't doing well with your diabetes care can make you even more depressed, resulting in a downward spiral of diabetes highs and emotional lows.

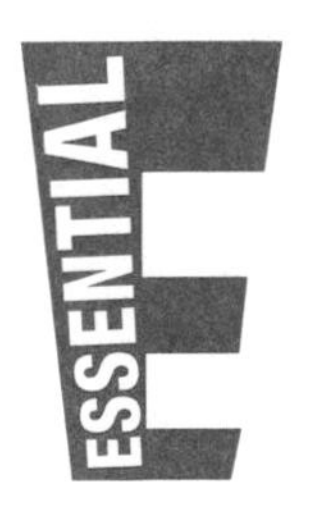

Diabetes can be a heavy load to carry, and depression seems to double that weight. Ignore either and they'll only get worse. You don't have to suffer in silence. Let your doctor know if you're experiencing signs of depression. Therapy or antidepressant medication may be options for you.

Weighty Issues

Women with type 1 diabetes may find their weight fluctuating with their insulin needs, which can be a source of frustration and may also take a toll on self-esteem, particularly in the teen years. For women with type 2 diabetes, who often have weight problems, negative body image is a prevalent problem.

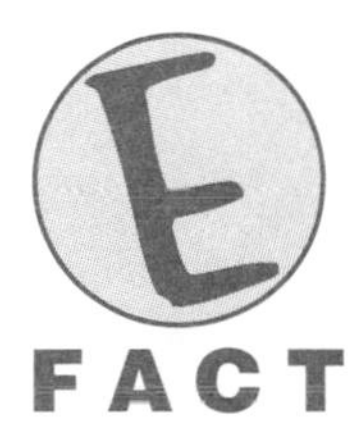

FACT

An April 2003 study in the *Journal of the American Medical Association* reported that women who watch twenty hours or more of television each week are more likely to experience obesity, diabetes, and other health risks. Researchers found that every two hours spent watching television was associated with a 14 percent increase in diabetes risk.

Aside from contributing to depression, a poor self-image can hinder your sex life and be a source of stress and anxiety. Living a fit and active lifestyle should not be identified with being supermodel skinny. Accepting yourself at any size is important to your physical and psychological well-being.

Sometimes weight problems can feel so insurmountable that women are hesitant to even take that first step forward for fear of failure. Soon they find themselves in an endless cycle of binging, bad feelings, and sky-high blood glucose levels. Consequently, self-esteem plummets along with diabetes control. Yes, weight loss can be hard, but you don't have to go it alone. Your doctor, registered dietitian, and diabetes care team are all there to help you succeed. See Chapter 13 for more information on the psychology of weight loss and sensible weight control.

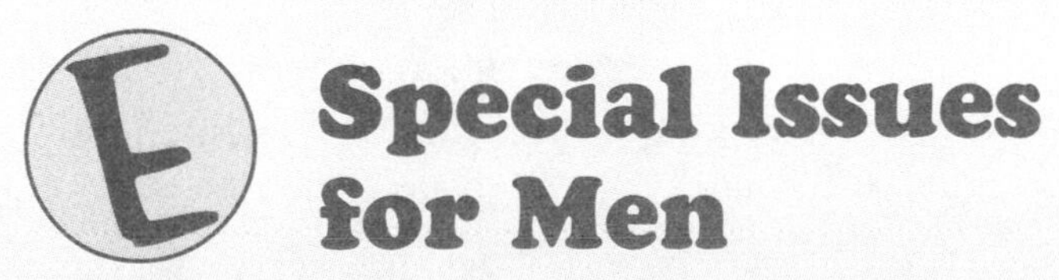

Chapter 19

Special Issues for Men

Men with diabetes face unique challenges of their own. You may be less apt to express any feelings of anxiety or depression you're facing while trying to come to terms with the disease, and one of the most prevalent complications in men with diabetes—impotence—is definitely an emotionally loaded issue. But while men face a higher risk of certain diabetic complications, they are more likely to report feeling in control of their diabetes and on top of their treatment, both big benefits in dealing with chronic disease.

At Puberty

The peak incidence of type 1 diabetes in boys is between the ages of twelve and fourteen, when puberty is up and running. The hormonal changes that accompany puberty actually increase insulin resistance in both boys and girls, which compounds the problem of insufficient insulin production in those with type 1 diabetes.

Insulin resistance may also be accompanied by increased resistance to growth hormone in boys, and poor control has the potential to impact the speed and course of the "growth spurt" that normally occurs at puberty.

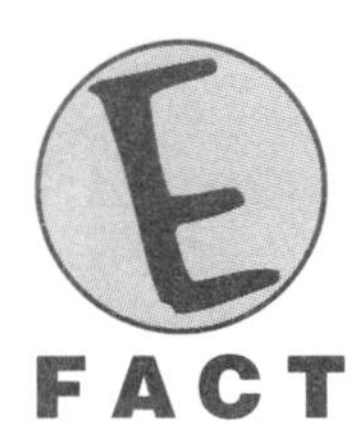

FACT

There are 7.8 million adult males with diabetes in the United States—that's 8.3 percent of all American men. An estimated one-third are not even aware that they have diabetes.

A Turbulent Time

Puberty is a time of separation from parents and a growing emphasis on social relationships—creating a separate social identity is paramount. Boys who may have depended on their parents for guidance on diabetes care may start taking more responsibility for their care. Likewise, parents must learn to hand over the reins of diabetes control, at least partially, to allow their child to mature emotionally as well as physically.

However, the social pressures of puberty can also push young men in the opposite direction, of ignoring their diabetes for the sake of being more like their peers. Drug and alcohol use—experimental or otherwise—can also become a problem during this time of life. American males ages 12 to 18 are statistically more likely to drink alcohol and take illicit drugs than girls of a similar age. In 2001, nearly 14 percent of eighth-grade boys and 23 percent of male high school seniors reported regular binge drinking.

Because alcohol can impair treatment judgment and trigger a potentially dangerous hypoglycemic episode, it's important that boys (and girls) with diabetes are educated about the special risks they face with alcohol and drug use. Even though "Just Say No" is good advice, realistically it may not be followed. Especially during adolescence, kids need to know what precautions are necessary if they do drink.

Changes in Testosterone Levels

Testosterone levels in men begin to decrease starting around age forty, eventually leading to what some have called "male menopause," or andropause, which brings with it an increased cardiovascular risk, loss of muscle and bone mass, and a waning libido. Other signs of declining testosterone can include lower sperm count, body hair loss, and even hot flashes.

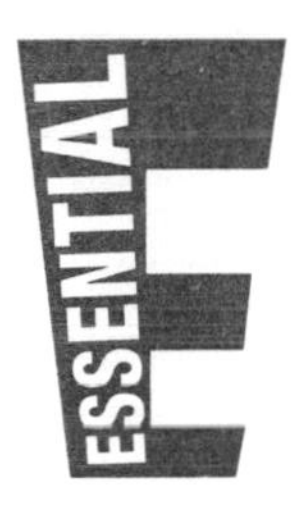

While low levels of testosterone are thought to be associated with central obesity, the opposite is true for women, in whom high levels of the hormone are tied to excess abdominal fat and insulin resistance.

Men with diabetes tend to have a lower than average testosterone level. The classic "apple-shaped" body of type 2 diabetes, also known variously as intraabdominal fat or central fat storage (or, in more familiar terms, beer belly), is associated with low testosterone levels in men. Also known as hypogonadism, this condition is also associated with high levels of circulating insulin (hyperinsulinemia) and increased insulin resistance. Low levels of the hormone are thought to affect glucose metabolism; some studies have linked improved glucose tolerance with testosterone replacement therapy.

HRT—Not Just for Women

Hormone replacement therapy, in the form of injections or a transdermal (through the skin) gel or patch, can be beneficial to many older men with low testosterone levels. The jury is still out on whether this therapy can slow or even prevent the onset of type 2 diabetes by inhibiting intraabdominal fat accumulation.

Sexuality and Impotence

Impotence—the failure to get or maintain an erection—is one of the most common and most distressing side effects of diabetes. Between 35 and 75 percent of men with diabetes have experienced impotence at some point since diagnosis. If you've had problems with erectile dysfunction (ED), you are not alone.

Some men delay getting treatment for ED because of embarrassment or self-consciousness, but ED can be the first sign of a more serious underlying diabetes complication, such as cardiovascular disease or neuropathy, so it's important not to ignore it or delay medical attention for the problem. Your doctor is quite used to dealing with impotence issues and has a variety of treatment options at his disposal.

What Causes ED

There are many possible causes of male impotence, ranging from surgery to smoking; the following are most likely to affect men with diabetes:

- **Medications.** Drugs such as high blood pressure medications, certain antidepressants, and tranquilizers can trigger episodes of impotence. Your doctor may be able to adjust your dosage or substitute another medication.
- **Neuropathy.** Nerve damage to the penis itself or to the autonomic nervous system may be the cause of ED.
- **Cardiovascular disease.** Clogged arteries, especially those which feed the corpora cavernosa (the spongy vascular tissue of the penis) can impair circulation enough to inhibit an erection.
- **Psychological issues.** Depression, anxiety, and stress related to diabetes management can inhibit sexual performance.

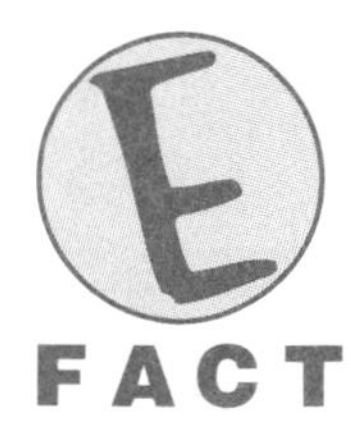

FACT

Smoking can contribute to erectile dysfunction by causing constriction of blood vessels, leading to hypertension. Nicotine also promotes the growth of artery-clogging cholesterol plaques, which also contribute to high blood pressure.

Treatment Options

There are a number of options available for treating ED, including medication, vacuum devices, surgery, and psychosocial therapy. The least-invasive nonpharmaceutical method of treatment is a mechanical vacuum device. A cylinder is placed over the length of the penis and a hand-operated vacuum pump is used to remove the air from the cylinder, creating a vacuum and pulling blood into the penis to create an erection. Once erection has been achieved, it is sustained with the use of a tension ring placed at the base of the penis.

The thought of a hypodermic syringe anywhere near your groin area might send shivers down your spine, but many men with ED caused by neuropathy can be helped with one of several drugs that are injected directly into the penis (papaverine hydrochloride; phentolamine; alprostadil, or Caverject) to dilate, or widen, blood vessels and cause an erection. Alprostadil is also available in a suppository (Medicated Urethral System for Injection, or MUSE) that can be inserted into the urethra, a more palatable choice for some men. Topical vasodilators (e.g., nitroglycerin ointment, minoxidil)—medications that are rubbed on the penis to improve blood flow—may also be an option, but reports of their success are mixed.

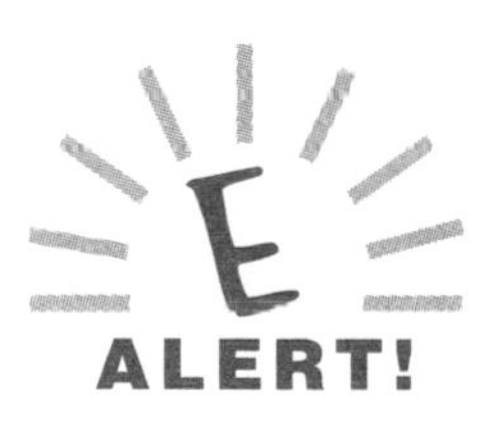

Men who use nitroglycerin ointment to treat ED should wear a condom during intercourse. Nitroglycerin is absorbed through the skin, including the vagina, and can cause a headache or other symptoms in your partner. Of course, wearing a condom is always recommended if you aren't involved in a long-term, monogamous relationship.

Viagra (sildenafil citrate) has helped millions of men with erectile dysfunction problems since its release in 1998. The drug is taken about an hour before sexual activity and works by enhancing the effects of nitric oxide on the body, which dilates blood vessels and acts as a smooth-muscle relaxant. This improves blood flow to the penis and facilitates an erection when sexual arousal occurs.

Several clinical studies have demonstrated that Viagra is well-tolerated by men with both type 1 and type 2 diabetes, and can help these men improve their erectile function significantly. One potential drawback is the need to take the drug sixty minutes before sex; if you're a spur-of-the-moment kind of guy you'll need a new strategy.

Two new drugs for ED—vardenafil and Cialis (tadalafil)—were still pending FDA market clearance for U.S. sale as of early 2003.

Insertion of a penile implant, or treatment and repair of arterial and venous damage related to ED, are more invasive options to treat impotence. Your doctor can discuss treatment options that are right for you.

If your impotence is rooted in depression, anxiety, or other emotional issues, your doctor may refer you to a counselor, psychiatrist, or psychologist for help in sorting through it all. A couples therapist may also be helpful for uncovering sources of marital tension.

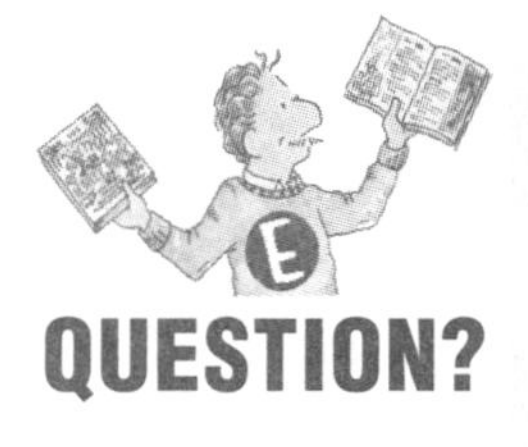
QUESTION?

I have diabetes and hypertension. Can sex make my heart condition worse?

Unless your heart is severely impaired (i.e., congestive heart failure), there is really very little risk of normal sexual activity triggering a heart attack. Halting all exercise—and sex—is probably one of the worst things for your hypertension. A chat with your doctor about your concerns will help you ease your mind about sex.

Diabetes and Fertility

Men with long-term, uncontrolled diabetes can suffer nerve damage that causes a condition known as *retrograde ejaculation*—where sperm is deposited into the urinary bladder instead of being ejaculated out the head of the penis. This happens because the small muscle that controls the passageway into the bladder becomes damaged and doesn't close as it should during climax, so sperm is rerouted into the bladder.

Some men may have reduced ejaculate as a result of this condition, while others may not ejaculate at all. The latter is referred to as "dry climax." Retrograde ejaculation can be a cause of male infertility, and if it is caused by neuropathy it cannot be surgically corrected at this point in time.

If you have symptoms of the condition, you should talk to your doctor about a referral to a urologist. Couples who have trouble conceiving due to retrograde ejaculation should see a fertility specialist. Assisted reproduction may be a possibility by retrieving sperm through a bladder-washing procedure and using it to artificially inseminate your partner.

Complications: Gender Bias?

While diabetes crosses all age, racial, and gender lines, it does seem to show some questionably preferential treatment to men in the distribution of certain diabetic complications. For example, the ADA reports that men diagnosed with diabetes before age thirty tend to develop retinopathy more rapidly than their female counterparts. And among people with diabetes, first heart attacks are more likely to be fatal in men than women.

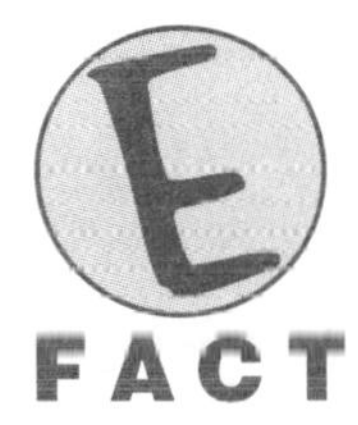

FACT

According to the ADA, amputation rates are 1.4 to 2.7 times higher in men than women. However, with proper preventative foot care and wound treatment, your risk drops dramatically.

Men with type 2 diabetes are more likely to develop coronary artery disease (CAD) than women with the disease and than their male counterparts without diabetes. They are also more likely to have additional CAD risk factors, such as high triglycerides, high blood pressure, and obesity.

How Men Cope

A ten-year study of gender differences in attitudes toward diabetes at the Johns Hopkins Diabetes Center found that men tended to have more positive attitudes toward and greater acceptance of their diabetes than women with the disease. Accordingly, they also tended to rate their quality of life higher. The study also found that men were more accepting of their treatment regimen, and were less likely to miss work or leisure activities due to their diabetes.

Perhaps reflecting traditional "woman as caretaker" gender roles, men with diabetes were also most satisfied with the level of emotional support they received from their wives or partners, who were more likely to accompany them to appointments and diabetes education classes than male partners or husbands of women with diabetes. Interestingly, while men with diabetes did not miss work or leisure activities, their wives were more likely to have to take time off attributed to their husband's disease, yet these women reportedly feeling less anxious about the long-term impact of the disease on their family than the husbands of women with diabetes.

Men in this study also reported more control over their diabetes in terms of lower HbA1c levels, better self-reported nutritional care and insulin compliance, and fewer complications than women have.

Men and Stress Management

But what about when things don't go right? Problems with erratic blood glucose levels and elusive control can cause stress levels to climb. This leads to a vicious cycle of control issues, as high stress produces high glucose levels, high blood pressure, and further anxiety about your ability to manage your disease.

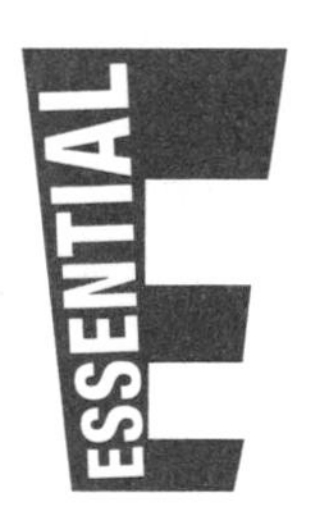

When things aren't going well with diabetes management, some men can take it as a sign of personal failure, or an affront to their masculinity, and the resulting stress can make the situation worse. Think of erratic blood glucose levels as a challenge rather than a fault. Use your health care team and your support system to figure out the mystery.

Studies have demonstrated that stress management training can improve long-term blood glucose control, thus reducing your risk of complications. They have also demonstrated that daily practice of stress management techniques by men with heart disease can slash their risk of cardiovascular incidents like surgery and heart attack in comparison with those who used exercise or standard therapy (medication and monitoring). For more on stress management and diabetes, see Chapter 20.

Chapter 20

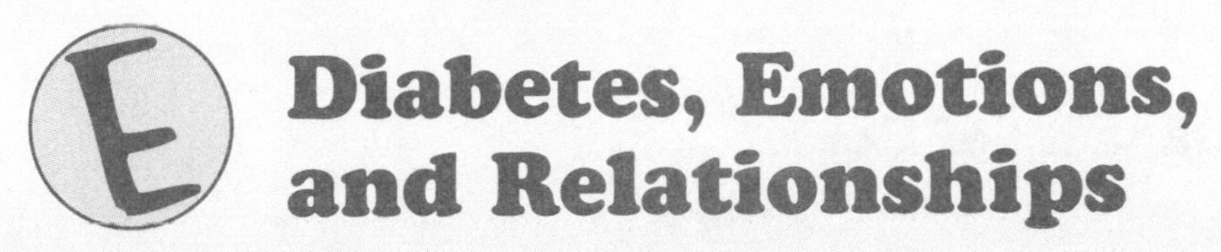

Diabetes, Emotions, and Relationships

In addition to blood sugar highs and lows, diabetes triggers emotional ups and downs that can be just as unpredictable and severe. And because the disease is life altering, it has a significant impact on not just the patient, but on everyone who lives with and cares for her or him. Preparing yourself for the emotional issues that diabetes brings can help you maintain your sanity and strengthen your relationships with others.

Dealing with Diagnosis

Dealing with a diabetes diagnosis has been compared to coping with the grief of death. Diagnosis marks the loss of life as you knew it. It's normal to grieve your old "healthy" life, even if you weren't feeling well before getting the diabetes label. Denial, anger, bargaining, depression, and acceptance are all part of the process.

The Dangers of Denial

The first of these can be the hardest and most damaging in diabetes. Many people chose to simply ignore that they have the disease, continuing on as if it didn't exist. The problem with this (non)coping approach is the long-term consequences of uncontrolled blood glucose. By the time they do come to terms with denial and are ready to treat their diabetes, serious complications may be on their way.

Some newly diagnosed patients will acknowledge their feelings of denial. Recognition is a good sign that in the back of your mind you know you must move forward. As long as you're willing to follow your doctor's orders for the time being, even if you haven't fully accepted the disease, denial is a normal part of the process.

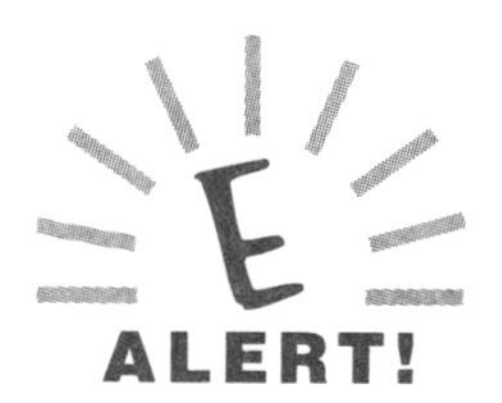

For patients who reject both the diagnosis and the treatment, the situation can become a dangerous one. Sometimes it takes a blood sugar emergency that lands them in the hospital for them to realize that they do, indeed, have diabetes.

Reaching acceptance can be a difficult, rocky road. Many people need the help of a therapist or counselor to get there. A health psychologist who has specialized training in the intricate psychological, biological, and social relationships between physical illness and mental health can be helpful in sorting through coping issues.

The Emotional Roller Coaster

Although acceptance is an important step in getting on track to diabetes control, it isn't a guarantee of ongoing inner peace. Periods of difficult control and high blood sugars can also bring devastating emotional lows, which can in turn make blood glucose levels rise even further and start a self-perpetuating cycle of physical and psychological deterioration. Learn to recognize the signs of emotional pitfalls like depression, anger, guilt, and stress so you can take the appropriate steps to stop this downward spiral before it starts.

Depression

Up to 20 percent of people with diabetes also suffer from depression. Occasional sadness, fear, and uncertainty are normal in diabetes, but when they start affecting your everyday enjoyment of life and interfering with proper self-care, they may be something more than just a passing emotional downturn.

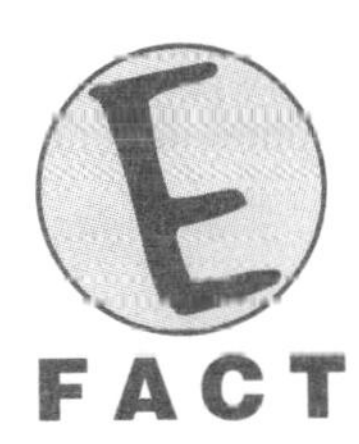

Signs of a depressive disorder include weight loss, insomnia or hypersomnia (too little or too much sleep), irritability or agitation, fatigue, feelings of guilt or worthlessness, inability to concentrate, and recurrent thoughts of death or suicide.

Depression can be treated with therapy and/or antidepressant medication, so there's no reason to suffer needlessly. Here are a few other strategies that may help you deal with depression:

- **Knowledge is power.** Fear of the unknown can feed your depression. If you haven't already, start educating yourself about your disease.
- **Seek support.** Draw on the experience and emotional comfort of your family, friends, spiritual community, health care team, and others with diabetes.
- **Keep perfection in perspective.** Reward your successes, big or small, and try to see your stumbles as learning experiences rather than failures.

- **Keep moving.** Try to push yourself to at least take a brisk walk daily. Exercise raises your endorphin levels, a natural mood booster.

Anger Management

You have diabetes and you're foot-stamping, wall-slamming, screaming, steaming mad about it. Now the question is, what do you do with all that pent-up hostility? Do you focus it on beating the snot out of that damn disease through aggressive diabetes control, or do you turn it outward at the world and push away your family and care providers in the process?

Anger is an understandable reaction to diabetes, and it can be a good motivational tool if used appropriately. However, if it's becoming a barrier to your care and your relationships with others, it's a problem.

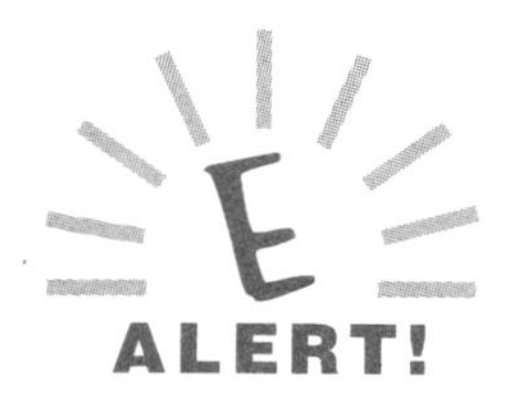

Anger is a common symptom of a blood sugar low. If you feel yourself getting angry for no good reason, it may be a sign you need to test your blood sugar. And if you live with someone with diabetes, try not to take anger personally when it occurs in connection with a low. Remind yourself that it's the diabetes talking, and move past any hurt feelings to help treat the hypoglycemia.

Feeling Guilty

It may not be rational, but it's perfectly normal to feel guilty about having diabetes. But now that you know it's normal, it's time to move on. You are not to blame for having diabetes, nor should you feel ashamed of your diagnosis. You've done nothing to deserve your disease; your genetic makeup and/or environmental factors have made you susceptible to it through no fault of your own.

Managing Stress

When you face a physically or psychologically stressful situation, your body starts a complex process of hormone release and reaction. The adrenal glands start to pump out cortisol, the hormone primarily responsible for our physiological "fight or flight" reaction to situations we perceive as dangerous. Cortisol signals the liver to start up glucose production to give the brain and central nervous system added energy, while signaling the fat and muscle tissues to slow their uptake. It also causes the release of fatty acids from fat tissues, which are needed for muscle fuel, and sends your blood pressure up.

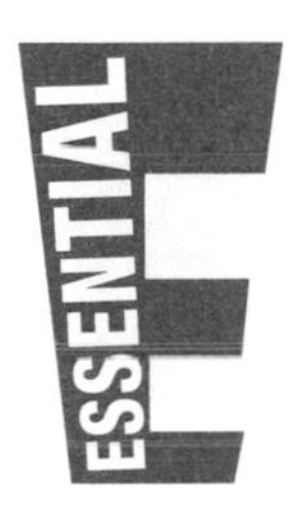

No one, and that means no one, has perfect diabetes management skills all the time. If you have an unforeseen high or low, don't take it as a sign of personal failure. Measure your success by your commitment to care. When a high or low happens, learn from the experience to prevent it the next time.

Stress also prompts the adrenal glands to release epinephrine, the hormone that provides the adrenaline rush of the "fight or flight" reaction. High levels of circulating cortisol and epinephrine promote insulin resistance in addition to ratcheting up blood glucose levels.

Since it increases blood pressure and spikes glucose levels, stress is obviously not the best medicine for diabetes control. And it's dangerous because it may distract you from controlling your diabetes as you become preoccupied with other issues.

The Physical Toll

When you're ill or suffer an injury, your body is stressed and you need to test more frequently. The same goes for times when you are mentally and emotionally under duress. Audited by the IRS? On double shifts at work? Taking final exams? Make sure you test glucose levels more often than usual.

Stress has also been associated with abdominal or visceral adiposity (that "apple" shape); it's unclear, though, whether stress causes a spare tire and the spare tire causes type 2.

Make a Change

Studies have shown that stress management programs can be extremely effective in improving psychological well-being and diabetes control. One 2002 Duke University study published in *Diabetes Care* found that just five sessions of stress management training lowered A1c levels an average of half a percentage point.

The Duke study involved a stress-training regimen of audiotape-led progressive muscle relaxation, cognitive and behavioral therapy (including guided imagery and deep-breathing exercises), and education on the mechanisms and health consequences of stress.

Other good stress management techniques include yoga, music or art therapy, and journaling. Anything that calms you and allows you to relax and release is a good stress management strategy.

Turning to a Support Group

For the same reason that diabetes camps are a huge boon to kids with type 1 diabetes, support groups are an absolutely invaluable resource for adults with diabetes. A support group offers patients a chance to compare treatment notes, to talk about emotional issues in living with the disease—even to air their gripes about the health care system. In addition to expanding your knowledge and fostering a sense of camaraderie, a support group is a good stress-release valve.

Your doctor's office and/or local hospital are good places to check on existing support groups. If you find that your community doesn't have one, ask your physician or diabetes educator about the possible interest level in a group among other patients. You may be able to set up one of your own.

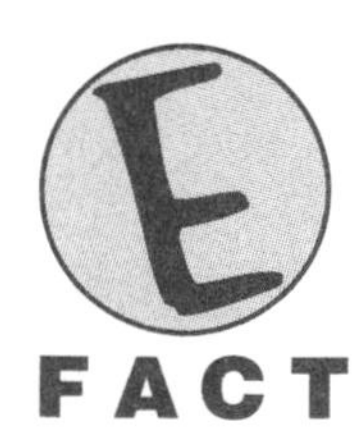

FACT

While physical stress like injury, illness, or trauma causes blood glucose levels to rise in both type 1 and type 2, mental stress consistently causes rises only in type 2 diabetes. Most people with type 1 diabetes will also have a rise in levels in conjunction with psychological stress, but some will actually experience a drop.

Around the World

Online communities for people with diabetes are plentiful and can be almost as—if not more—supportive and informative than real-time groups. There's input from Pennsylvania to Paris, with participants from all walks of life and a broad range of experience with diabetes and diabetic complications. On the other hand, you may get inaccurate medical information from people who either don't know better or who are trying to sell some miracle cure.

The "miracle" workers can be taken care of with the firm hand of a good moderator. As long as you take what you read with a grain of salt, you certainly stand more to gain than you can lose. And the beauty of an online support group is that it is there all day and all night for your questions, vents, and gripes.

The Dating Game

Single with diabetes? You may feel like every encounter is a blind date as you consider whether or not to "tell" about your diabetes. Or you may screen your potential partners by specifically mentioning the *D* word. There's no reason to treat your diabetes as a skeleton in the closet or a state secret, but some people feel more comfortable sharing their disease after they've laid the foundation for a relationship. The bottom line is, you should do what feels right to you.

Intimacy Issues

When things get intimate, they can also get a little weird. What if you go low and pass out in the heat of passion? Or what if your partner gets tangled up in your infusion set? Having a sexual encounter of the strange kind is the worst nightmare of many single people living with diabetes.

Making love with a partner you trust can alleviate much of the tension you might feel about your first time together. And what seems mortifying now is usually good for a laugh together later. The worst-case scenario rarely happens. Don't obsess over the "coulds" to the point where they become a major preoccupation.

For Spouses and Significant Others

When your partner is handed a diabetes diagnosis, so are you. Get on board with diabetes care right off the bat. You can and should attend diabetes education classes to learn more about the disease and how to treat it. If you do the grocery shopping and/or cooking in your household, you should absolutely attend the meeting your partner has with a registered dietitian. And if your partner feels comfortable with it, go along on doctor's visits as well. Two sets of ears are always better than one.

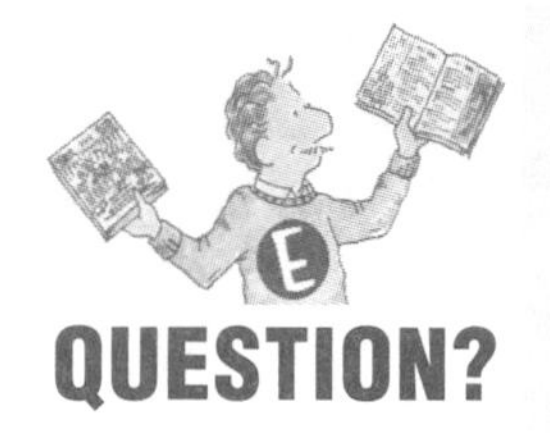

QUESTION?

My husband has had problems in the bedroom ever since he was diagnosed with type 2 diabetes. Is this part of the disease?
If your husband is newly diagnosed, he may be struggling to come to terms with diabetes. Depression, anxiety, and anger are all common emotions following diagnosis of a chronic illness, and could temporarily affect his libido. However, diabetes-associated impotence is quite common. For more on the subject, see Chapter 19.

Try (and it can be hard) not to become the diabetes patrol. Think of what it would be like to go through life listening to the following:

- "Are you sure you can eat that?"
- "Do you *really* think you should have that?"
- "Don't you think you should do something about that reading?"

Communicate openly and honestly with your partner about how you can help when things aren't going right, before they go astray. That way you know in advance the most effective way to assist.

Helping Those Who Don't Help Themselves

Perhaps you're reading this book because you're more interested in diabetes control than your significant other–the one with the disease–is. Maybe your partner hasn't come to terms with his diagnosis yet, or maybe he's depressed or disheartened and has stopped trying. You can read and learn until you're blue in the face, and you may even be able to nag your partner into a few extra glucose checks or a more appropriate meal. But you can't control his diabetes for him. Remember this if you remember nothing else. Your mental health and emotional well-being are just as important as your partner's, and you can save yourself countless hours of head-banging frustration if you detach enough to realize that he is the pilot of the diabetes ship.

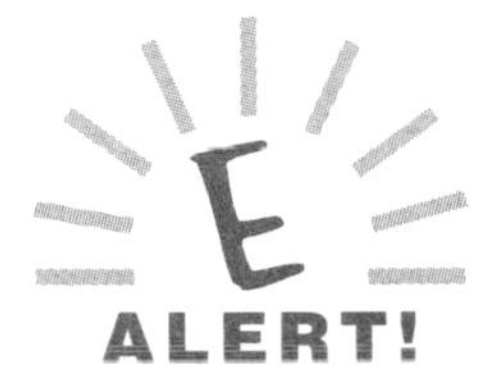

Support your spouse or partner, but keep in mind that she, and not you, is in charge of taking care of her diabetes. This means being there for her if she asks for help, offering to go to the doctor's appointments with her, but not pushing the issue, and not eating things under her nose that she can't have.

At the same time, you don't want to go too far in the other direction and make it easier for your partner to get away with screwing up his control by going along with his program. Accepting his excuses about why that extra piece of pie just had to be eaten or nodding your head when she says she's going to cut back her insulin to drop a few pounds is not being supportive. It's called "enabling," and spouses and family members of alcoholics do it all the time. Don't let yourself become part of the problem, or validate bad behaviors.

Caring for Kids with Diabetes

Diabetes affects the entire family—beyond the lifestyle adjustments a family is faced with, there is fear, guilt, jealousy, anger, and other emotions to come to terms with. Both the parent/child and the sibling relationship can face difficult challenges that require empathy, discipline, and flexibility to work through and beyond.

Whether a parent or child has diabetes, the whole family can benefit from diabetes education classes. Even small children can learn more about the disease through age-appropriate books. It's easy to feel isolated when you have diabetes, and involvement of the family goes a long way toward creating a caring and supportive environment that makes control easier.

To Love and Not Overprotect

When your child has diabetes, he or she has more boundaries than others, and it can be easy to fall into the trap of making them tighter than necessary. Letting your fears overtake your child's normal social development is not healthy for either of you. Kids need to be kids—to participate in sports, to go to birthday parties, to spend the day at the beach with friends, and to go to school dances and football games.

Follow the "first do no harm" motto of the medical profession and take the least-invasive route when making decisions on what your child can and cannot do, based on your child's age, responsibility, and level of competence with her or his own diabetes care. And if you must say no, let your child know the reasoning behind the decision. "Because I said so" is not a good explanation, and will not help to make boundaries clearer to your son or daughter.

As your child grows and takes a greater deal of control over her own care, you may find yourself feeling strangely unneeded. Remember that your adolescent is forming her own identity and needs the autonomy to make some of her own treatment decisions and take over more of her day-to-day management. You do need to remain a partner in her care, however. Asking if she's changed her infusion set or helping her check her glucose if she doesn't look well is still your responsibility as parent and care partner.

Sibling Issues

One child has diabetes and the other doesn't. How do you balance one child's restrictions with the other's relative lack of them? And how do you balance out all the necessary time and attention given to caring for your child with diabetes in the eyes of your child who doesn't require constant oversight? Parenting can be even more of a challenge when you're caring for a child with diabetes and a child without it. You feel as if you're constantly saying "no" to both of them.

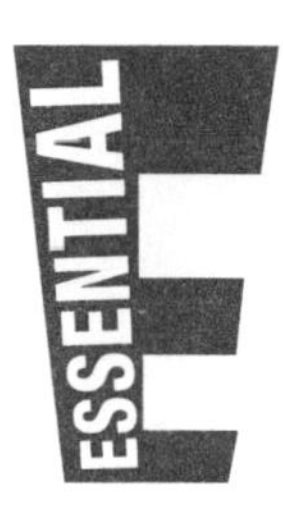

Caregivers need care, too. While it gets easier with practice and age, it's emotionally exhausting to stand guard over your child day in and day out. Arrange for backup care for your child at least once a month and get out and enjoy yourself. You might also check out the availability of support groups for parents of children with diabetes in your area as both a sounding board and shoulder to lean on.

Try to make life as normal as possible for both of them. Healthy eating habits and activity should be a family goal. The sibling without diabetes should be educated about the other's special needs, something that will probably come naturally in the course of everyday home life. However, you need to make it clear that only parents or another responsible adult are to treat the disease, as some children may try to "help" with a younger sibling and unknowingly place them in danger. Your child with diabetes needs to feel safe about his care, and also guilt-free about having special requirements associated with the disease.

At the same time, don't let your child get manipulative with his disease. Using it as an excuse to get out of chores or tasks, or playing the "poor me" card to get you to agree to special privileges should not be allowed, particularly when it's at the expense of your other child. Being a parent of a dual-diagnosis (one with, one without) household can be a challenge, but you're up to the task. To learn more about parenting a child with diabetes, see Chapter 17.

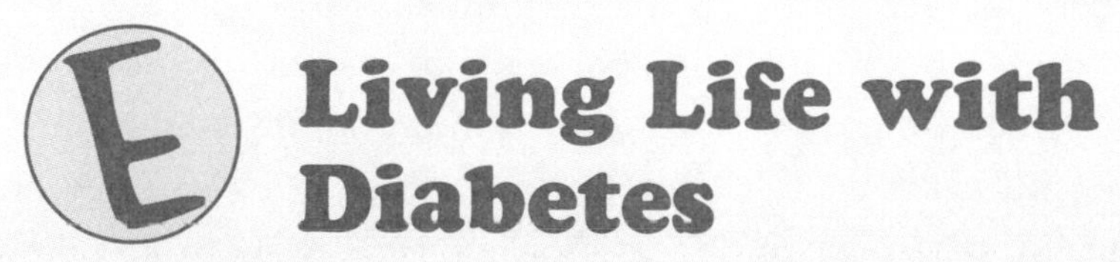

Chapter 21

Living Life with Diabetes

In theory, there's nothing you can't do now that you couldn't do before you had diabetes. But in practice, you will have to make some lifestyle adjustments to manage your disease well. It's kind of like that old joke about the violin—"Doctor, will I ever be able to play the violin again? Yes? But I couldn't play it before. . . ." You may actually be able to do things bigger and better than you could before your diagnosis.

Diabetes at Home

Even though you're the one with the diabetes diagnosis, your whole family needs to make some adjustments to living with the disease. A healthful lifestyle promoting good blood glucose control is the best defense against diabetic complications. And the good news is that it's a great prescription for everyone around you as well.

Don't try to go it alone. The changes that diabetes brings to the dinner table can be positive ones for the entire family, particularly if your diet before now has been less than stellar. Exercise is also a healthy choice for the whole family, both physically and on a psychological level—the family that plays together stays together.

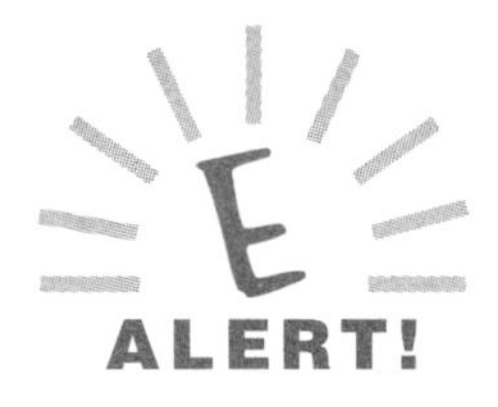

While kids should be able to enjoy the occasional treat that isn't regularly on your meal plan (read: Ding Dongs and Oreos), stocking up on junk food isn't healthy for you or them. You don't need the temptation and they will be better off with more balanced fare. Limit "treats" to special occasions like Halloween or birthdays.

You may hear the "why should we all have to suffer?" defense as you encourage your family to join you on your new and healthier lifestyle. Step back and assess what might be causing that reaction. Fear of giving up the familiar is one possibility. You might also be asking them to do too much too fast, particularly if you were stuck in a pizza, Chinese takeout, and McDonald's routine.

Start Out Slowly

Try limiting restaurant food to once a week and encouraging healthier menu choices. Instead of mandating "no junk food" off the bat, allow one selection of their choosing to be kept in a cabinet you don't frequent. Above all, work to provide lots of healthy, fresh, and good-tasting alternatives so the change is perceived as a positive one.

If your family members have a favorite food that's a no-no for you, only keep it on hand if you're sure it won't be calling you from the cupboard. Remember, you are not an ogre for requesting that potato chips, Moon Pies, and Lucky Charms be kept out of the pantry. No matter what degree of pouting and resistance you face from your spouse or children, stand firm. Bypassing these treats won't harm their health; having them could very well hurt yours.

Make Your Needs Known

It's easy to get discouraged and depressed when others don't seem to be meeting your needs or don't even seem to be aware that you have them. Stop those feelings before they start by laying out exactly what you need from the people around you.

If you find you don't have enough time to exercise as you should because of child care responsibilities, tell your spouse it's essential to your health to get some assistance. If your significant other keeps making you all the things you shouldn't be eating, give her some guidance. Go with her on the next grocery shopping expedition, or, better yet, take her with you on your next appointment with the CDE or dietitian. Don't expect your family and friends to be mind readers. Assume they know next to nothing about your new lifestyle needs, and educate them accordingly.

Making Your Home Diabetes-Friendly

There's more to treatment success than whipping the pantry into shape. The first is keeping a frequent watch on where your glucose levels are. One way to encourage yourself is to have several meters available where you'll use them—in the kitchen, by your bed, in your gym bag. If you're often testing at night, there's at least one model on the market with a glow-in-the-dark faceplate for easier testing. You can use your kitchen timer or alarm clock to remind you to take any postprandial blood sugar checks. Keep several blood sugar logs with your meters so you remember to record your results, or carry a pocket-sized "master log" with you to keep everything in one place.

Home safety is also an issue. If you don't have one already, get a sharps disposal bin. Even if you don't use insulin, you should still have one for your lancets. If you have a small child with type 1 diabetes, you will have to be twice as vigilant about toddler-proofing your home, particularly the kitchen. Keep the cupboards and pantry closed and locked (or fastened with child safety latches) to avoid any surreptitious snacking.

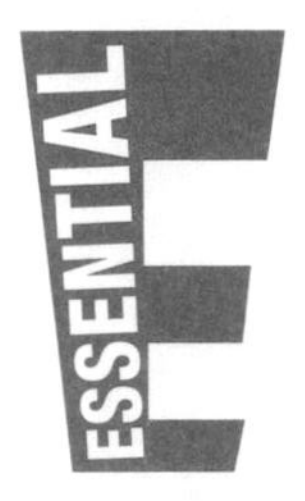

Stress is a well-known offender in causing blood glucose levels to rise, particularly in patients with type 2 diabetes. Yoga, progressive relaxation, massage therapy, exercise, and meditation are just a few ways to de-stress. Talk therapy, either one-on-one with a counselor or in a support group, can also be extremely helpful.

Diabetes at Work

If you are employed outside the home, you may need to make some adjustments in your daily work routine to accommodate good treatment habits. There's probably no job out there that is perfectly suited for diabetes, but there are some employment situations that are more difficult than others. Working a job where you're on your feet all day, where it's difficult to take a break to test your blood sugar, where your shifts are unpredictable, or where you are exposed to extreme heat or cold can make control hard.

You may be faced with some tough choices as you try to make your job compatible with your new life. The legal protections offered by the Americans with Disabilities Act will help to a degree, but even with that, you may find yourself in a position where your job is working against your diabetes management. If this is the case, you do have options:

- Talk to your doctor about adjustments to your treatment. Could a new medication or insulin regimen help?
- Talk to your boss or manager about adjustments to your work schedule or other accommodations. Is a transfer possible or preferred? Could a shift change be in order?
- Explore your options both inside and outside of your company. If you've been contemplating a career change or return to school, maybe now is the time to get moving.

Third-shift work and swing-shift work (where your work shifts are switched on a regular basis) are particularly hard on diabetes management, which strives for balance. If you must work these types of hours, you need to stay in close contact with your diabetes care team to keep on top of problems as they arise and make any necessary medication and insulin adjustments.

Discrimination: What the Law Says

The Americans with Disabilities Act (ADA), passed in 1992, prevents your employer from discriminating against you solely on the basis of your diabetes, and it requires that employers make "reasonable accommodations" to allow you to check your blood glucose and treat yourself as needed. Under the act, a disability is a record of "physical or mental impairment that substantially limits one or more of the major life activities" of an individual. The ADA applies to all employers with fifteen or more employees.

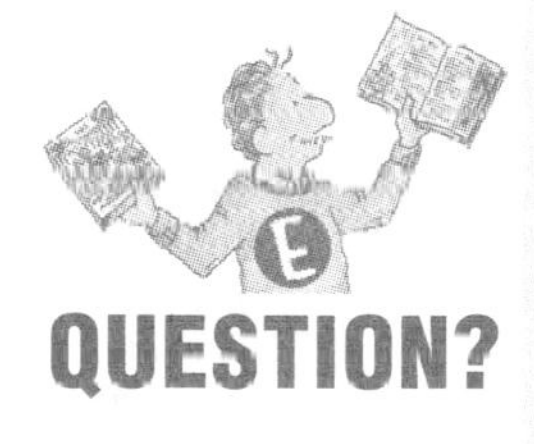

I don't consider myself disabled just because I have diabetes. Am I sending the wrong message to my employer and coworkers if I claim protection under the ADA?
The ADA was designed to cover a broad range of Americans who may experience discrimination in the workplace due to health issues, and is your best protection for fair treatment on the job. Don't toss it aside based on semantics alone. When you invoke your rights under the ADA, you ensure you are judged on your abilities rather than your disease.

Providing a small refrigerator for your supplies, giving you short breaks to check glucose, and adjusting your work shift if it causes control problems would all fall under the scope of reasonable accommodation in most cases. If the accommodation is said to provide "undue hardship" on the employer (usually in terms of financial resources), it may not be required. Generally speaking, the majority of accommodations that would be required for diabetes would not be considered an undue hardship under the ADA for most organizations. However, you should consult a lawyer specializing in disability law if you have specific questions about your situation and employer.

Your employer cannot deny you health benefits; under the ADA you are entitled to the same health insurance, disability, and other benefits as other employees in your workplace. And if your spouse or child develops diabetes and you carry insurance for your family through your employer, you are covered by these same provisions.

Job Hunting

Looking for a job? The ADA protects you against discrimination here as well. Know that questions about your health in an interview are illegal, and so is withdrawing a job offer based on your diabetes alone. If your diabetes is disclosed during a preemployment physical, your prospective employer cannot use it as a reason to deny you employment as long as reasonable accommodations can be made for you. Of course, going for the head wine-taster job at the local vineyard isn't a good idea; there may be certain positions that require activities you just can't perform or that can't be "reasonably accommodated." In addition, you may be legally unable to obtain licensure for certain positions like commercial truck driving, depending on the state you live in. However, if you already work one of these positions and develop diabetes, your employer must offer you another suitable vacant position within the company (as long as you are qualified to perform the new job). The ADA also prevents your employer from denying you a promotion based on your diabetes.

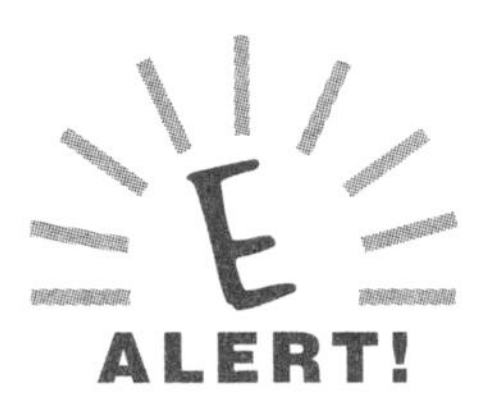

If based on the employer's words or actions you have any reason to believe you were discriminated against because of your disease, contact the Equal Employment Opportunity Commission ADA hotline at 1-800-669-3302.

Workplace Accommodations

There are many benefits to providing a working environment that accommodates people with diabetes and other chronic illnesses.

Employee satisfaction, better retention rate, fewer sick days, and lower disability payout are just a few good motivations. It also takes money and resources to train employees, and if you are a good worker, it makes sense for your employer to do what it can to retain you.

If the people in your workplace don't seem to know a lot about diabetes, take the opportunity to teach them. Let your human resources director know about the Diabetes at Work program (*www.diabetesatwork.org*), which educates employers about diabetes and offers advice on instituting screening and wellness programs designed to reduce diabetic complications. The American Diabetes Association is also an excellent source of information for your employer.

To Tell or Not to Tell

Telling others can be hard. You may be afraid of job discrimination. And sometimes it can be difficult admitting you need help. However, you can't claim protection under the ADA if you don't let your employer know about your condition and ask for accommodation assistance. If you're inexplicably missing work or taking longer or more frequent breaks without permission, you may very well lose your job.

There are several good reasons to let your coworkers in on your diabetes. First and foremost, people around you need to know what to do in case of a blood sugar emergency. Second, it's an excellent opportunity to spread awareness of the disease and perhaps educate them in the process. And finally, if your employer has allowed you extra breaks and other accommodations to check your glucose levels and treat yourself, letting coworkers in on the reason why can prevent feelings of ill will.

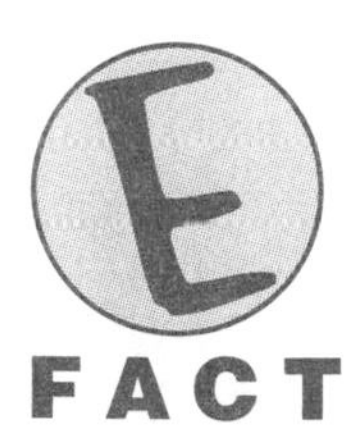

FACT

Under the Americans with Disabilities Act, your employer must maintain your confidentiality about your health condition, disclosing it to others only on a "need to know" basis (for example, if you work in a manufacturing environment where a company nurse is on staff, she would be informed of your condition so she could treat you appropriately).

Eat, Drink, and Be Wary

Birthday parties, family reunions, wedding receptions, holiday office gatherings—any event where food and drink play a starring role is a potential danger zone without the right preparation. If you know the fare will be high in fat or sugar-rich, bring along a healthy dish (your hostess will probably appreciate the contribution). Having a small snack at home before the event can help to blunt your appetite against too many temptations.

Don't forget that dancing is exercise. Check your glucose levels if you've been out on the dance floor for a while to ensure they aren't dropping too low. If food won't be available at all times during the party, bring a snack with you to fuel up. A nondiet soda or juice from the bar can help to treat a low if you're caught without glucose tablets.

If you decide to enjoy beer, wine, or a mixed drink, use caution and make sure you have a friend with you who can recognize the signs of a low and treat them accordingly. See Chapter 14 for more on avoiding lows when drinking.

Behind the Wheel

Always test before you drive, and if you're low, don't drive. Blood glucose levels below 70 mg/dl should be treated appropriately, and a safe blood sugar level should be attained before getting back behind the wheel. If you start to experience symptoms of hypoglycemia while you are driving, pull over immediately to test and treat. A low impairs your judgment and can cause you to lose consciousness. Like alcohol and falling asleep at the wheel, low blood sugars can easily result in a traffic fatality.

Licensing Issues

For people with well-controlled diabetes and a good driving record, maintaining a noncommercial driver's license shouldn't be an issue. State law governs regulations for driver's licenses, and in some cases your license may have medical restrictions (particularly if you are on insulin). In addition, if you have type 1 diabetes or take insulin for your type 2 diabetes, you may have your license suspended if you experience a hypoglycemic episode. In many states, your doctor is required to report you to the department of motor vehicles if he feels it is unsafe for you to drive due to your diabetes. If your diabetes is not well controlled, if you experience hypoglycemic unawareness, or if you have frequent lows, it may not be safe for you to drive a motor vehicle.

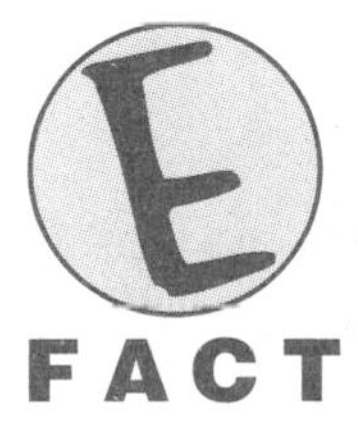

FACT

In the mid-1990s, the Federal Aviation Administration overturned a blanket ban on small-aircraft private pilot licenses for people who take insulin for their diabetes. These license applications are now handled on a case-by-case basis, evaluating each individual's specific medical situation.

Commercial licenses (CDLs) generally have much stricter regulations, again governed by state. In many states, taking insulin is grounds to have your commercial license revoked or not issued. The American Diabetes Association has been active in advocating the creation of a system that evaluates CDL applications on a case-by-case basis instead of with a blanket ban. Your state motor vehicle bureau can answer specific questions about the licensing laws in your area and how they apply to intrastate commercial truck driving as well.

On a Road Trip

The minivan, the open road, passing cornfields, roadside diners, the hourly "are we there yet?" question, the carsick baby. Ahhh—the pleasures of the family road trip. Taking a trip by car brings its own unique set of challenges to people living with diabetes. Prolonged sitting, road fatigue, truck stop dining, and should-have-turned-left-at-the-last-exit-but-won't-ask-for-directions syndrome are just a few of the roadblocks you may have to overcome.

Stop and stretch often to get your circulation going and cut fatigue. It's a good idea to check your glucose levels at each rest stop as well. Again, pack snacks just in case you get waylaid or don't count on the next restaurant being quite so far. A cooler is an excellent idea if you'll be traveling long stretches of remote highways. A cell phone is also essential for rural travel in case a breakdown leaves you stranded or you have a medical emergency.

Make sure all insulin, testing kits, and medication are stored someplace that won't get excessively hot or cold. Trunks, glove compartments, and dashboards are all bad spots to keep your supplies. If you're traveling in hot weather and you stop for a food or road break, do not leave your supplies and/or medication in the car unless you have a cooler to store them in. On a 73-degree day, in just ten minutes temperatures can reach 100 and higher in a car with the windows rolled up, which is bound to make your insulin go bad and possibly damage your meter and other equipment.

Be Prepared

Whether you're going by plane, train, or automobile, there are some basics you should carry with you at all times (as carry-on items) along with your toothbrush and clean underwear. These include:

- A first-aid kit, including antibiotic ointment and bandages
- Extra medication and insulin
- Blood glucose meter with double test strips, alcohol swabs, and lancets
- Extra batteries for your meter
- Emergency supply of fast-acting glucose
- Extra pump supplies (if applicable)
- Plenty of snacks, including fast-acting carbs

Always travel with twice the amount of medication and/or insulin you would normally require for the time you'll be gone. The same goes for blood glucose testing supplies. If you are delayed for weather or any other unexpected reason, your foresight will save you a lot of scrambling about trying to get a prescription filled in an unfamiliar place.

A sturdy, watertight supply case is a must for anyone who travels frequently. For those who take insulin, a case that is well padded and insulated to keep vials or pens at their proper temperature is also important.

Travel Tips for the Wise

Vacations and business travel can present some unique control challenges and safety issues. Don't travel completely alone unless you have to. In case of an emergency, a trusted friend, spouse, or companion will be invaluable, particularly if you're in a foreign country. If you're a free spirit and like to fly solo, make sure you always carry your basic medical information (i.e., name, diagnosis, medication, physician contact) on your person, and wear your medical ID prominently.

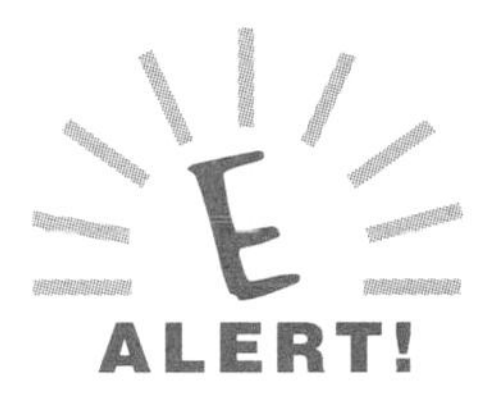

Cruises are notorious for lavish buffets and total indulgence, but that doesn't mean you have to miss the boat. There are a growing number of cruise packages designed just for people with diabetes—with healthy and delicious cuisine, diabetes education, and plenty of fun in the sun built in to the itinerary. Talk to your travel agent, or see the travel resources in Appendix A.

Leisure Travelers

How many times have you returned from a vacation to feel more exhausted and burned out than before you left? Try to lose the "hurry up and have fun—we're paying for this!" attitude and take a trip that involves actual rest and relaxation.

If you're traveling for leisure, try to throw strict schedules (except for those involving food and medication) out the window. Stress can drive your blood glucose levels up and put a damper on your fun. Don't overplan your days, leave room for flexibility, and enjoy just being in a new environment or culture.

Business Travelers

Travel for business may throw some unexpected restrictions into your routine. A meeting with a client or an all-day workshop, and suddenly you find yourself behind schedule and going low. You can't work effectively if you don't take care of yourself, so excuse yourself if things run longer than expected. In fact, the best approach is probably to mention a departure time as soon as your meeting begins, and stick to it. If you feel uncomfortable mentioning that you need a time-out to eat or take medication due to your diabetes, then tell your client or colleague you have a dinner or lunch meeting to make (which is entirely true). You can also continue your business over a meal if you feel comfortable doing so.

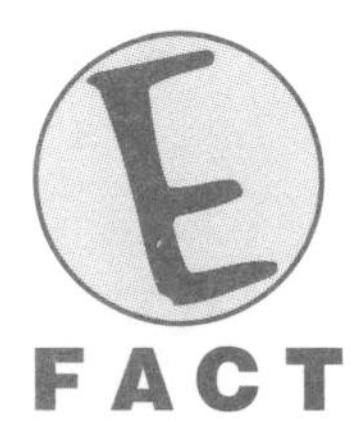

FACT

Many airlines offer meals for special diets (kosher, diabetic, low-sodium, vegetarian, and so on). Request a special meal when you make your reservation, but pack an extra snack just in case it turns out to be something less than appetizing.

Air Travel and Medical Devices

In the last few years, air travel security measures have changed significantly in the United States and abroad. Because having diabetes necessitates traveling with medical sharps, there are some extra steps you may need to take to ensure you have easy access to your insulin and testing supplies while flying.

- **Insulin.** Keep all original packaging and paperwork that come with your insulin so you can present the original printed pharmaceutical label for the medication at the airport security checkpoint. The same applies for Glucagon kits. Syringes will be allowed past security only if the accompanying medication is properly labeled.
- **Meters.** The FAA will allow glucose meters and lancets in suitcases or carry-on baggage as long as meters are clearly marked with the manufacturer and/or brand name. Lancets should be capped and properly stored with the meter.
- **Pumps.** If you wear an insulin pump, inform airport security personnel and request that they visually inspect it rather than removing it. Again, have insulin documentation with you. If screeners insist you remove your insulin pump, ask to speak with a security checkpoint supervisor.

Allow plenty of extra time for getting through airport security. You may want to plan on an extra thirty to sixty minutes in addition to whatever your airline is advising for advance arrival time. This will give you breathing room if airport personnel need to check out your medical supplies. And always call the airline you'll be traveling with first to find out their specific security policies for the flight itself.

If you have problems with improper treatment or discrimination when traveling by air, call the Transportation Security Administration (TSA) hotline at 1-866-289-9673. Complaints may be filed in writing with the Department of Transportation's Office of Civil Aviation Security: Office of Civil Aviation Security (ACS-1), 800 Independence Ave., S.W., Room 1030, Washington, DC 20591. You can also contact the American Diabetes Association for assistance at 703-549-1500, ext. 2108. The ADA works with the FAA and TSA on an ongoing basis to improve diabetes awareness among airport security personnel.

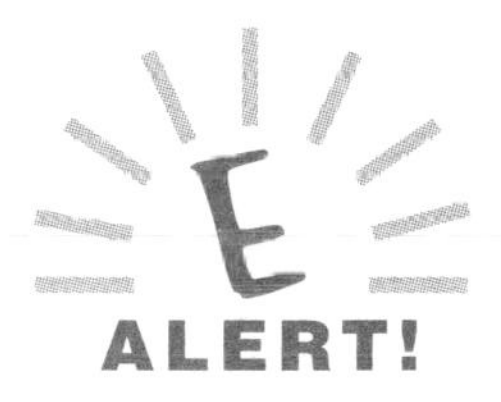

If you have peripheral vascular disease, you run the risk of developing deep-vein thrombosis (DVT, or blood clotting) if you remain immobile for long periods of time. When you take a long flight or drive, be sure to get up and stretch your legs periodically. Wearing elastic compression stockings (i.e., support hose) may also be beneficial.

Adjusting Insulin and Time Zones

International travel requires some extra planning, particularly if you take insulin. In addition to the usual jet lag, you have to keep on schedule with your medication. In general, the easiest and most practical approach is to take insulin on track with meals in the "new" time zone you're traveling in (or are en route to). However, you should always consult your doctor about appropriate adjustments to insulin and medication before you travel, as his advice may vary based on the type of insulin you take, the distance you are traveling, and other factors specific to your situation.

Staying Well Abroad

To stay healthy and safe while traveling in a foreign country, you should make sure you can communicate your needs adequately and are well supplied for the journey. Some tips:

- **Get your shots.** Before you go, make sure any required immunizations are up to date.
- **Learn the language.** If you don't speak the native tongue, make sure you have a guidebook to help you with basic medical phrases like "I need a doctor" and "I have diabetes."
- **Have your papers in order.** Keep your doctor's name and phone number along with your written insulin schedule on you at all times, and, as always, wear your medical identification.
- **Drink water.** If the water is questionable, drink bottled (and hold the ice in any canned and bottled beverages you order) to avoid diarrhea or more serious illnesses.
- **Keep a food supply.** Make sure you have a stash of nonperishable snacks like peanut butter and crackers, canned fruit juice, raisins, dried apricots, nutrition bars, and other foods that keep well and will serve as a mini-meal should your plans be interrupted.

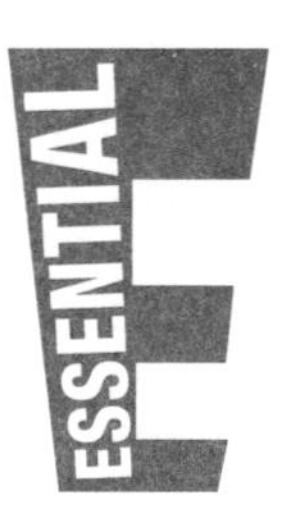

A number of diabetes drugs may cause photosensitivity (increased skin sensitivity to the sun) in those who use them. To minimize your risk, wear a brimmed hat and sunscreen with an SPF of 35 or higher for all exposed skin. Long sleeves and pants legs also increase protection.

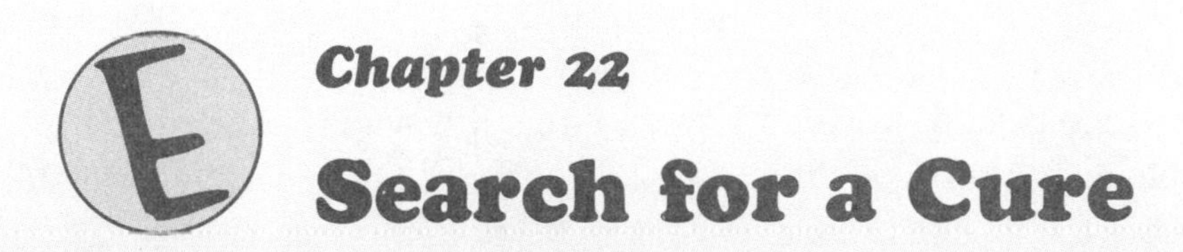

Chapter 22
Search for a Cure

Diabetes is, at present, an incurable disease. Although type 2 diabetes can be well controlled to the point of normal or near-normal blood glucose levels, once you have it, it's a lifelong companion. While type 1 diabetes can conceivably be "cured" with a pancreas or islet transplant, both of these procedures currently require a lifelong regimen of immunosuppressive drugs. Still, enormous strides in genetics, transplantation techniques, and stem cell research have brought a cure closer than ever.

A Short History

Diabetes was a death sentence for thousands of years until the discovery and isolation of insulin in 1921 provided the first groundbreaking step toward a cure. Before Sir Frederick Banting and Charles Best isolated the hormone, and colleagues J.J.R. Macleod and J.B. Collip helped purify and produce it for human use, the only treatment for diabetes was a near-starvation diet that resulted in slow wasting and eventual death.

Once insulin provided a way to treat the symptoms of diabetes, the challenge in the years that have followed has been to find a way to restore the insulin-producing capacity of the pancreas.

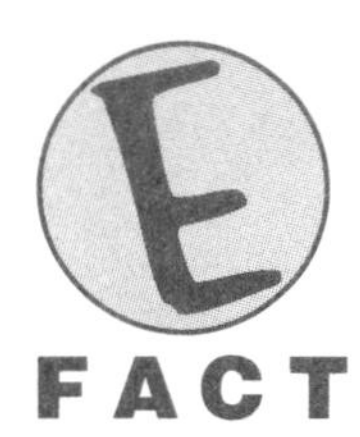

FACT

Sir Frederick Banting, codiscoverer of insulin, began treating one of his first and most famous patients in 1922. Elizabeth Hughes, the daughter of New York Governor Charles Evans Hughes, weighed only 45 pounds when Banting began treating her with twice-daily injections of insulin. She recovered rapidly, becoming a national medical miracle and living until age seventy-three.

Genetic Discoveries

Deciphering the genetic code behind the regulation of insulin production is one of the keys to finding the cure for diabetes. In 2002, researchers at Joslin Diabetes Center in Boston reported that they had isolated and cloned the third and what is believed to be final gene behind insulin production. These three genes—PDX-1, Neuro-D1, and RIPE3b1 factor—work together to trigger insulin production in the beta cells of the pancreas. Both PDX-1 and Neuro-D1 have been associated with maturity-onset diabetes in the young (MODY). When either of these two genes is missing, the pancreas and/or beta cells fail to develop normally, resulting in type 1 diabetes.

Researchers are now using this knowledge to try to find a way to coax stem cells, the building blocks of the human body, to develop into insulin-producing beta cells and possibly lead to a cure for diabetes. Stem cell research is covered in greater detail later in this chapter.

Unlocking the Beta Cell

Beta cells are the insulin-secreting cells of the pancreas. They are contained within islets (or islets of Langerhans)—cell clusters found within the pancreas. Islets are responsible for producing glucagon (alpha cells), insulin (beta cells), and somatostatin (delta cells). Destruction of the insulin-producing beta cells results in type 1 diabetes, so the search for a cure has focused on finding a healthy replacement for these cells.

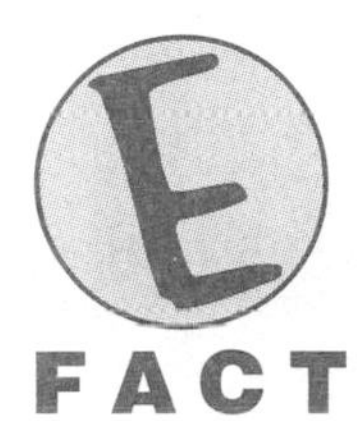

FACT

Islet transplantation has been under development since 1976, when the first successful animal islet transplant was performed by Dr. Paul Lacy, a JDRF (Juvenile Diabetes Research Foundation)-funded researcher.

Transplants

One way to replace beta cell function and re-establish insulin independence is through a pancreas transplant. The procedure, however, is relatively rare. Only 163 pancreas transplants were performed in the United States in 2001, due to both a lack of available organs and the risk of potential toxicity of the immunosuppressive drugs required post-transplant. More common is the combined kidney-pancreas transplant, which 885 patients underwent in that same year. And according to the United Network for Organ Sharing (UNOS), 305 more patients received a PAK, or pancreas after kidney transplant, in 2001.

The reason both kidney-pancreas transplants and pancreas after kidney transplants are more common than pancreas-only transplants is the strict regimen of immunosuppressive drugs required for any transplant procedure. People with type 1 diabetes are already at risk for autoimmune problems and are more prone to infections, so further suppression of the immune system is risky.

However, because of the high incidence of chronic kidney failure in people with diabetes, the need for a kidney transplant is higher than in the general population. If a patient has developed end-stage renal disease and requires a kidney transplant and accompanying immunosuppressive therapy anyway, the logic is that doing a simultaneous pancreas transplant typically can't hurt and can only help in most cases.

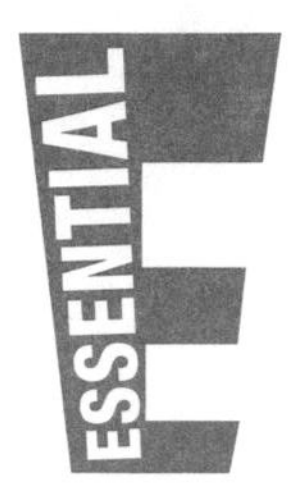

Organs for transplant are still in much greater demand than supply. According to the Juvenile Diabetes Research Foundation (JDRF), there are about 1 million people in the United States with type 1 diabetes, but only about 2,000 donor pancreases are available each year for transplants.

The Edmonton Protocol

Since only 2 percent of the pancreas is composed of islets, a transplant of islets only is less invasive and has a much quicker recovery time than a full pancreas transplant. The Edmonton Protocol is a procedure for transplanting pancreatic islets into people with type 1 diabetes in an effort to reverse their diabetes. The procedure, which was developed at the University of Alberta (Canada), involves infusing healthy, insulin-producing islets into the portal vein through a catheter. They are carried through the bloodstream to the liver, where they attach and begin functioning. The Edmonton Protocol also involves treating the patient post-transplant with a specialized steroid-free immunosuppressive cocktail of the drugs daclizumab, tacrolimus, and sirolimus.

Dr. James Shapiro, the lead researcher behind the Edmonton Protocol, first published the protocol and its remarkable success rates in the *New England Journal of Medicine* in 2000. Since that time, clinical trials of the procedure have expanded rapidly and are taking place in research institutions throughout North America. At the time of publication of this book, researchers were reporting one-year success rates (as measured by insulin independence) of over 80 percent, a significant advance over dismal pre-Edmonton rates of less than 10 percent.

One of the major obstacles in widespread application of islet transplantation is an inadequate supply of islets. The Edmonton protocol involves infusion of a larger volume of freshly harvested islets than previous islet transplantation methods used. In fact, two donated cadaver pancreases are required for each islet transplant procedure. Given the shortage of donated organs in the United States and abroad, this is where stem cell research may hold a prominent role in the search for a cure. In addition, there are numerous complications that could possibly occur as a result of islet transplantation, including bleeding, blood clots, gallbladder injury, worsening of lipids, elevation of blood pressure, worsening of kidney function, acne, and mouth ulcers. Some of these complications are due to the procedure, while others are a result of the drugs being used.

Stem Cell Research

Stem cells are uncoded, "generic" cells from which virtually all tissues of the body develop. These blank slates can be programmed into any organ, tissue type, or blood cell with the right set of genetic influences, or expressions.

The stem cells that have shown the most promise in diabetes research are those derived from in vitro fertilization (IVF), which are more commonly known as *embryonic stem cells.* These cells have the unique capacity to become any type of cell, tissue, or organ as they mature and develop, yet they cannot themselves develop into a full human being. The feature that makes them most useful as a source for islets is that they can replicate themselves while remaining in an immature, or "undifferentiated" state, thus offering a potentially unlimited source of cells for organ transplantation.

Growing Stem Cells

Stem cells are grown, or cultured, in a laboratory. The cells grow in a culture dish treated with a growth medium. The culture is sometimes treated with embryonic skin cells from mice, called feeder cells, to prevent the stem cells from dividing (or differentiating) and to provide nutrients to the culture. Because of the possibility of virus transmittal between human stem cells and feeder cells, researchers have been attempting to move away from this method of culturing cells.

Once cells have been cultured many times over, usually over the course of six months or longer, and have continued to reproduce without dividing or differentiating, they are said to be an established stem cell line, the basic materials that researchers use for specific experimentation.

A Matter of Controversy

Of course, stem cell research has become a political, social, and ethical hot button issue in the past decade because of the nature of embryonic stem cells. These cells are derived from a blastocyst–a hollow ball of cells from a four- or five-day-old embryo derived from an egg fertilized outside of the body in an IVF clinic. The current status of federally funded research in the United States does allow study of embryonic cells, but only those currently available from a limited number of existing cell lines.

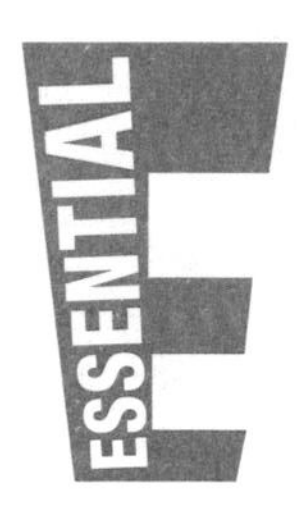

Adult stem cells are a less controversial but, thus far, less productive area of diabetes research. These undifferentiated cells come from bone marrow or other areas of the body and act as a built-in first-aid kit, repairing tissue injury in the body. Scientists have also found that some of these adult stem cells can be coaxed into new tissues and organs.

Building a Better Pancreas

One goal of current diabetes research is to find a way to "close the loop" on glucose monitoring and insulin treatment. In laymen's terms, this means a device that will monitor glucose levels and deliver insulin in response without any required operator intervention. Basically, this device would act as an artificial pancreas.

One closed-loop system currently in development is the long-term sensor system, or LTSS (Medtronic MiniMed), which is a surgically placed system that links an implantable long-term glucose sensor with an implantable insulin pump. The glucose sensor is implanted in the superior vena cava, a blood vessel near the heart, where it continuously monitors blood glucose levels. The sensor then transmits the information to the insulin pump, implanted in the abdomen, which in turn infuses the correct amount of insulin. The unit is programmed with a small computerized device that uses radio frequency signals to send messages to the pump.

The LTSS requires an insulin refill every several months, which can be performed in a simple outpatient procedure using a syringe device. Safety mechanisms prevent the insulin from releasing unless it locks on to the correct port of the pump.

Another less-invasive version of a closed-loop system, in development by insulin pump manufacturer Disetronic, uses an external approach instead of an implantable one. The unit consists of a blood glucose sensor that adheres to the skin, an insulin pump, and a small computer that analyzes glucose levels and signals the pump to infuse insulin in correct amounts in response.

Both Medtronic MiniMed and Disetronic have their artificial pancreas products in clinical trials, and predict bringing them to the market by 2007.

Clinical Trials

Clinical trials are scientific research studies that examine different aspects of a disease or medical condition or evaluate new drugs and other treatments. By participating in a clinical trial, you can get free access to new therapies not yet available to others. However, you also take any risks associated with an unproven treatment.

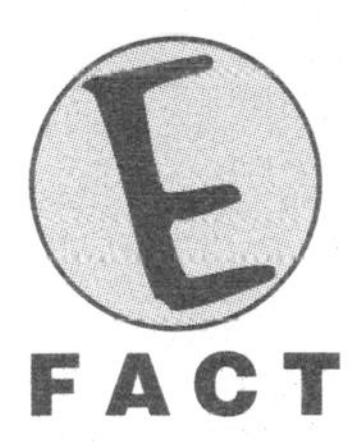

FACT

Clinical trials of new drugs fall into four different "phase" categories. Phase 1 studies are initial, small-scale trials that help establish a safe dose and determine side effects. Phase 2 uses a larger study population at the dose established in phase 1 to determine the efficacy of the drug, and phase 3 and 4 studies compare the new drug with existing treatments for the same condition or illness.

All clinical trials have to meet guidelines outlined by both the National Institutes of Health (NIH) and the U.S. Food and Drug Administration (FDA). They also must meet the specific criteria of the institution that sponsors the research. A governing body known as an *institutional review board* (IRB) oversees the study design and protocols to ensure it meets specific ethical, clinical, and safety standards.

Informed Consent

It's important to note that when you agree to participate in a clinical trial, you may not necessarily receive the treatment that the study is evaluating. Depending on the design of the study, you may be chosen to be part of a control group (a group of study subjects that does not receive the therapy being tested in order to serve as a baseline for comparison), or you may receive a placebo (an inactive substance that is sometimes administered to half of the study group, to measure the effectiveness of the treatment against a control).

Learning all of the potential ins and outs of a clinical trial is part of receiving informed consent on the study. Because the treatments examined in clinical trials are still experimental, informed consent is an important aspect of meeting the ethical guidelines of scientific study.

If you're interested in participating in a clinical trial, your first step is to check and see what is available. The government Web site *www.clinicaltrials.gov* has a database of NIH-sponsored trials. If you live near a research institution or university, you can also check on available clinical trials there. Eligibility requirements will vary with each study.

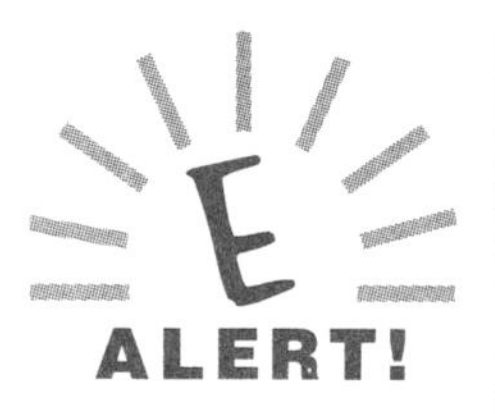

It bears repeating yet again that the onset of type 2 diabetes can be dramatically delayed or even halted with relatively minor lifestyle changes. If you are at risk for type 2 diabetes but have not developed the condition yet, the best thing you can do for your health is to get on an exercise and healthy dietary program.

Diabetes Prevention Program (DPP)

DPP was a landmark national study of 3,234 people with prediabetes (impaired glucose tolerance). The study found that diet and exercise slashed the risk of developing type 2 diabetes by 58 percent. The amount of exercise involved was just thirty minutes of moderate-intensity walking or similar workout routine daily, and the average weight loss was 5 to 7 percent of body weight. The study also found that subjects with prediabetes who were given treatment with metformin reduced their risk of getting type 2 diabetes by 31 percent.

Diabetes Prevention Trial—Type 1 (DPT-1)

DPT-1 is a large-scale national study involving over 80,000 subjects who are considered "at risk" for developing the disease (i.e., first- and second-degree relatives of people with type 1 diabetes). The trial was still under way as of the publication of this book. However, one arm of the study, which looked at the effectiveness of low-dose insulin injections in preventing or delaying the onset of type 1 diabetes in individuals considered high risk (i.e., greater than 50 percent chance of developing diabetes) was completed in 2002. Unfortunately, the DPT-1 found that insulin shots were an ineffective preventative measure at the dose tested in high-risk individuals.

Phase two of the DPT-1 is now exploring the possibility of whether oral insulin can prevent type 1 diabetes in people at moderate risk (i.e., 25 to 50 percent) of developing type 1 diabetes within five years. Regardless of the outcome of this trial, the knowledge gained in this landmark study will increase the current understanding of the disease and advance the search for a cure.

Advocacy Groups

You literally have the power of millions on your side in the fight against diabetes. Along with the 17 million Americans living with this disease, high-clout national advocacy organizations like the American Diabetes Association and the Juvenile Diabetes Research Foundation fight each day for diabetes rights, treatment advances, and a permanent solution to the disease—a cure.

Diabetes research also has many friends on Capitol Hill, including senators and representatives who have personally been touched by the disease. By adding your voice to the call for increases in research funding, both through your vote and with your support of advocacy and education in your community, you take the cause a little bit further. Yes, diabetes is a powerful enemy, but with strength in numbers, the fight can be won.

Appendix A

Additional Resources

General Diabetes Information

About Diabetes at About.com, hosted by Paula Ford-Martin (your author), *http://diabetes.about.com*

Dr. Ian Blumer's Practical Guide to Diabetes, *www.ianblumer.com*

Joslin Diabetes Center, *www.joslin.org*

National Institute of Diabetes and Digestive and Kidney Diseases (NIDDK), the National Institutes of Health, *www.niddk.nih.gov*

Rick Mendosa's Diabetes Directory *www.mendosa.com*

Kids and Diabetes

Children with Diabetes, *www.childrenwithdiabetes.org*

Countdown for Kids, *www.jdrf.org/kids/cfk/index.html*

Diabetes Camping Association, *www.diabetescamps.org*

Juvenile Diabetes Research Foundation, *www.jdrf.org*

The ADA Wizdom Youth Zone, *www.diabetes.org/wizdom*

Teens, Adolescents, and Young Adults

Reality Check, *www.realitycheck.org.au*

Teen Talk at Diabetes Station, *www.diabetesportal.com/teentalk*

Gestational Diabetes (GDM)

About Pregnancy at About.com, with Robin Elise Weiss *http://pregnancy.about.com*

National Institute of Child Health and Human Development (NICHD), *www.nichd.nih.gov*

Finding Your Health Care Team

American Academy of Dermatology (AAD), 888-462-DERM, *www.aad.org*

American Academy of Neurology (AAN), 800-879-1960, *www.aan.com*

American Academy of Ophthalmology (AAO), 314-991-4100, *www.aao.org*

American Association of Clinical Endocrinologists (AACE), *www.aace.com*

American Association of Diabetes Educators (AADE), 800-338-3633, *www.aadenet.org*

American Podiatric Medical Association (APMA), 800-ASK-APMA, *www.apma.org*

Food and Nutrition

About Diabetes Recipe Box, *http://diabetes.about.com/library/blrecipes/blrecipemain.htm*

About Nutrition at About.com, hosted by Rick Hall, MS, RD, *http://nutrition.about.com*

American Dietetic Association, *www.eatright.org*

Cinnamon Hearts, hosted by food writer Marilyn Helton (who also lives with type 2 diabetes), *www.cinnamonhearts.com*

The Diabetic Gourmet magazine, *www.diabeticgourmet.com*

University of Sydney GI Web site, *www.glycemicindex.com*

Travel with Diabetes

CDC Travelers' Health, *www.cdc.gov/travel*

Diabetes Travel Information, *www.diabetes-travel.co.uk*

Dynasty Specialty Group Cruises (in conjunction with Joslin Diabetes Center), *www.diabetesworkshopcruises.com*

Society for Accessible Travel and Hospitality, *www.sath.org*

Advocacy Organizations

American Diabetes Association (ADA), *www.diabetes.org*

Canadian Diabetes Association (CDA), *www.diabetes.ca*

Diabetes Australia (DA), *www.diabetesaustralia.com.au*

Diabetes UK, *www.diabetes.org.uk*

International Diabetes Federation (IDF), *www.idf.org*

Juvenile Diabetes Research Foundation (JDRF), *www.jdrf.org*

Patient Assistance Programs

The Pharmaceutical Research and Manufacturers of America (PhRMA), *www.helpingpatients.org*

Support Groups

About Diabetes Forum, *http://diabetes.about.com/mpboards.htm*

Diabetes Station, *www.diabetesstation.org*

Positive Diabetic Pregnancy, *http://groups.yahoo.com/group/PositiveDiabeticPregnancy*

Search for a Cure

The Diabetes Research Institute, *www.drinet.org*

The Insulin-Free Times, *www.insulinfreetimes.org/current.htm*

Juvenile Diabetes Research Foundation (JDRF), *www.jdrf.org*

Appendix B

Glucose Conversion Charts

HbA1c to Mean Daily Plasma Glucose Conversion

Use the following chart to figure out how your A1c results convert to an average daily blood glucose reading.

A1c percentile	Average plasma glucose level in mg/dL	Average plasma glucose level in mmol/l
12.0 percent	345	19.5
11.0 percent	310	17.5
10.0 percent	275	15.5
9.0 percent	240	13.5
8.0 percent	205	11.5
7.0 percent	170	9.5
6.0 percent	135	7.5
5.0 percent	100	5.5
4.0 percent	65	3.5

Recommended hemoglobin A1c (HbA1c) goal from the American Association of Clinical Endocrinologists is ≤6.5 percent; the American Diabetes Association recommends <7 percent.

Conversion calculation based on Rohlfing CL, Wiedmeyer HM, Little RR, England JD, Tennill A, Goldstein DE: "Defining the relationship between plasma glucose and HbA_{1c}: analysis of glucose profiles and HbA_{1c} in the Diabetes Control and Complications Trial." *Diabetes Care* 25:275–278, 2002.

Other Blood Glucose Conversions

To convert between mg/dl and mmol/l:

1 mmol/l = 18 mg/dl
1 mg/dl = .055 mmol/l

To convert from plasma to whole blood:

Plasma readings run about 15 percent higher than whole-blood readings.
Equation conversion factor: plasma = whole blood × 1.12

Appendix C

Preventative Care Guidelines

Regular preventative care is especially important when you have diabetes. The following chart is based on the recommended preventative care testing guidelines from both the ADA and the AACE. **Please remember that these are guidelines only, and you may need more frequent and/or additional diagnostic testing based on your particular medical history and diabetic complications.** For example, if you have known kidney problems, your physician will test your microalbumin levels more frequently, and if you have coronary artery disease, your regular visits may include additional cardiovascular assessment. Your diabetes care provider should discuss testing recommendations specific to your needs.

	Quarterly Exams	Annual Exams	Each Office Visit
Blood pressure and pulse			X
Height and weight			X
*Cholesterol (lipid panel)		X	
Comprehensive dilated-eye exam		X	
Foot exam			X
HbA1c	X		
**Microalbumin		X	

*Children two and older who have normal lipid profiles and low-risk status may have cholesterol testing every five years according to ADA guidelines. Low-risk adults (LDL <100 mg/dl, HDL >60 mg/dl, triglycerides <150) can be tested every two years.

**The ADA recommends that microalbumin screening start at diagnosis in patients with type 2 diabetes, and five years after diagnosis in patients with type 1.

Sources: Standards of Medical Care for Patients with Diabetes Mellitus, *Diabetes Care,* 2003 Jan. 26: 33S-50S. AACE Diabetes Guidelines, *Endocr Pract.*, 2002; 8 (Suppl 1).

Index

H

I

J, K

U, V

W

Everything® Kids' Hidden Pictures Book ($9.95 CAN)
Everything® Kids' Joke Book
Everything® Kids' Knock Knock Book ($9.95 CAN)
Everything® Kids' Math Puzzles Book
Everything® Kids' Mazes Book
Everything® Kids' Money Book ($11.95 CAN)
Everything® Kids' Monsters Book
Everything® Kids' Nature Book ($11.95 CAN)
Everything® Kids' Puzzle Book
Everything® Kids' Riddles & Brain Teasers Book
Everything® Kids' Science Experiments Book
Everything® Kids' Soccer Book
Everything® Kids' Travel Activity Book

KIDS' STORY BOOKS

Everything® Bedtime Story Book
Everything® Bible Stories Book
Everything® Fairy Tales Book
Everything® Mother Goose Book

LANGUAGE

Everything® Conversational Japanese Book (with CD), $19.95 ($31.95 CAN)
Everything® Inglés Book
Everything® French Phrase Book, $9.95 ($15.95 CAN)
Everything® Learning French Book
Everything® Learning German Book
Everything® Learning Italian Book
Everything® Learning Latin Book
Everything® Learning Spanish Book
Everything® Sign Language Book
Everything® Spanish Phrase Book, $9.95 ($15.95 CAN)
Everything® Spanish Verb Book, $9.95 ($15.95 CAN)

MUSIC

Everything® Drums Book (with CD), $19.95 ($31.95 CAN)
Everything® Guitar Book
Everything® Home Recording Book
Everything® Playing Piano and Keyboards Book
Everything® Rock & Blues Guitar Book (with CD), $19.95 ($31.95 CAN)
Everything® Songwriting Book

NEW AGE

Everything® Astrology Book
Everything® Divining the Future Book
Everything® Dreams Book
Everything® Ghost Book
Everything® Love Signs Book, $9.95 ($15.95 CAN)
Everything® Meditation Book
Everything® Numerology Book
Everything® Paganism Book
Everything® Palmistry Book
Everything® Psychic Book
Everything® Spells & Charms Book
Everything® Tarot Book
Everything® Wicca and Witchcraft Book

PARENTING

Everything® Baby Names Book
Everything® Baby Shower Book
Everything® Baby's First Food Book
Everything® Baby's First Year Book
Everything® Birthing Book
Everything® Breastfeeding Book
Everything® Father-to-Be Book
Everything® Get Ready for Baby Book
Everything® Getting Pregnant Book
Everything® Homeschooling Book
Everything® Parent's Guide to Children with Asperger's Syndrome
Everything® Parent's Guide to Children with Autism
Everything® Parent's Guide to Children with Dyslexia
Everything® Parent's Guide to Positive Discipline
Everything® Parent's Guide to Raising a Successful Child
Everything® Parenting a Teenager Book
Everything® Potty Training Book, $9.95 ($15.95 CAN)
Everything® Pregnancy Book, 2nd Ed.
Everything® Pregnancy Fitness Book
Everything® Pregnancy Nutrition Book
Everything® Pregnancy Organizer, $15.00 ($22.95 CAN)
Everything® Toddler Book
Everything® Tween Book

PERSONAL FINANCE

Everything® Budgeting Book
Everything® Get Out of Debt Book
Everything® Get Rich Book
Everything® Homebuying Book, 2nd Ed.
Everything® Homeselling Book
Everything® Investing Book
Everything® Money Book
Everything® Mutual Funds Book
Everything® Online Business Book
Everything® Personal Finance Book
Everything® Personal Finance in Your 20s & 30s Book
Everything® Real Estate Investing Book
Everything® Wills & Estate Planning Book

PETS

Everything® Cat Book
Everything® Dog Book
Everything® Dog Training and Tricks Book
Everything® Golden Retriever Book
Everything® Horse Book
Everything® Labrador Retriever Book
Everything® Poodle Book
Everything® Puppy Book
Everything® Rottweiler Book
Everything® Tropical Fish Book

REFERENCE

Everything® Astronomy Book
Everything® Car Care Book
Everything® Christmas Book, $15.00 ($21.95 CAN)
Everything® Classical Mythology Book
Everything® Einstein Book
Everything® Etiquette Book
Everything® Great Thinkers Book
Everything® Philosophy Book
Everything® Psychology Book
Everything® Shakespeare Book
Everything® Tall Tales, Legends, & Other Outrageous Lies Book
Everything® Toasts Book
Everything® Trivia Book
Everything® Weather Book

RELIGION

Everything® Angels Book
Everything® Bible Book
Everything® Buddhism Book
Everything® Catholicism Book
Everything® Christianity Book
Everything® Jewish History & Heritage Book

All Everything® books are priced at $12.95 or $14.95, unless otherwise stated. Prices subject to change without notice.
Canadian prices range from $11.95–$31.95, and are subject to change without notice.